Atlas of Orthopaedic Surgical Approaches

Edited by

C. L. Colton MB, BS, LRCP, FRCS, FRCS(Ed.)
Consultant Trauma and Orthopaedic Surgeon; Clinical Teacher, Nottingham University Hospital, UK

A. J. Hall MB, BS, LRCP, FRCS
Consultant Orthopaedic Surgeon, Charing Cross Hospital, London; Regional Adviser in Orthopaedics NW Thames, London, UK

The editors wish to express their sincerest thanks to the artist,
Joanna Cameron, BA (Hons), MMAA

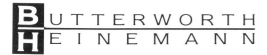

BUTTERWORTH
HEINEMANN

Butterworth-Heinemann Ltd
Linacre House, Jordan Hill, Oxford OX2 8DP

 A member of the Reed Elsevier group

OXFORD   LONDON   BOSTON
MUNICH   NEW DELHI   SINGAPORE   SYDNEY
TOKYO   TORONTO   WELLINGTON

First published 1991
First published as a paperback edition 1993

© Butterworth-Heinemann Ltd 1991

British Library Cataloguing in Publication Data
Atlas of orthopaedic surgical approaches
    1. Medicine. Orthopaedics. Surgery
    I. Colton, Christopher L. (Christopher Lewis)   II. Hall,
    A. J. (Anthony John)
    617.3

ISBN 0 7506 1702 0

Library of Congress Cataloguing in Publication Data
Atlas of orthopaedic surgical approaches/edited by
    C. L. Colton, A. J. Hall
    p. cm.
    Includes index; bibliographical references
    ISBN 0 7506 1702 0
    1. Orthopaedic surgery – atlases   I. Colton, Christopher
    L.   II. Hall, A. J. (Anthony John)
    [DNLM: 1. Orthopaedics – atlases   2. Surgery, operatives
    – atlases   WE 17 A880633]
    RD731.A89   1991   90–12794
    617.3–dc20   CIP

Cover illustration by Joanna Cameron

Printed in Great Britain at the University Press, Cambridge

Atlas of Orthopaedic Surgical Approaches

Foreword

The word 'atlas' derives from the name of the Greek god who upheld the pillars of the universe. While this present volume cannot bear quite so massive a burden, it can certainly support orthopaedic surgeons in their slightly less daunting task. It is, indeed, remarkable how much material has been encompassed in a relatively small space. This is partly because the editors have resisted the temptation to include the familiar preliminary chapters on basic principles, which hardly anybody reads, and those supplementary chapters on complications, which they read only with trepidation.

It required courage, as well as skill and hard work, to produce a book which is not lacking in recent rivals. But this courage has been rewarded, for few of the comparable publications can equal the clarity of its language or the elegance of the line drawings; the standard of both is consistently high. Moreover, all the approaches which an orthopaedic surgeon needs to know, or wants to know, have been covered, and covered well, in the 13 chapters which the book contains. There are also 13 contributors, but this is not a one-to-one relationship, for some chapters have more than one author and some authors have more than one chapter. But, though the authors disclaim any attempts to homogenize the text, differences of style and presentation are nowhere obtrusive. Editorial conferences and guidelines may well have helped to achieve this harmony, but a decisive factor must surely be that all the contributors are distinguished surgeons and their manifest practicality illuminates the text.

Some chapters seem to be better than others, but this is inevitable and may simply reflect my personal prejudices. I leave it to critics to court friendship by listing the chapters they like most, or to invite enmity by their omissions. Suffice it to say that no chapter falls below the high standard which the editors have set and that none fails to give clear practical guidance; editors and publishers all deserve congratulation on a fine production. I only wish this book had existed when I was training. Confronted with a difficult list I would have approached the operating theatre with more confidence and left it with more satisfaction.

A Graham Apley MB BS FRCS FRCS Ed (Hon)

Preface

This work arose from a perceived need for a comprehensive and authoritative compendium of most of those approaches required by the orthopaedic surgeon. The aim was to produce a work with an informative text supported by simple line diagrams. From the outset anatomical accuracy has been the prime consideration in the illustrations.

The work is aimed at the surgical trainee undertaking orthopaedic procedures, and surgical postgraduate examinees and their teachers who may need to update their confidence with unfamiliar approaches.

This is unashamedly a multi-contributor work and as a deliberate editorial policy no great effort has been made to 'homogenize' the text. The choice of the international body of authors has been based on their individual acknowledged expertise.

The reader will appreciate that in those regions of greater structural complexity a larger proportion of the section has been devoted to anatomical considerations than in others. The chapter on the spine is an exception as the related anatomy is of such complexity that only those structures particularly vulnerable have been highlighted. The reader should consult more detailed texts for additional anatomical information.

As the book has evolved through its production phase, surgical technology has advanced in some areas of the world making certain approaches redundant but it will be appreciated that in other geographical regions the more traditional surgical concepts still apply.

Contributors

N. J. Barton FRCS
Department of Hand Surgery, Nottingham University Hospital, UK

R. Birch MChir, FRCS
Orthopaedic Surgeon to St Mary's Hospital and Royal National
Orthopaedic Hospital, London, UK

C. L. Colton FRCS, FRCS(Ed)
Consultant Trauma and Orthopaedic Surgeon; Clinical Teacher,
Nottingham University Hospital, UK

J. R. Davey MD
Assistant Professor, Division of Orthopaedic Surgery, Toronto Western
Hospital, Canada

Alan E. Freeland MD
Professor, Department of Orthopedic Surgery, University of
Mississippi Medical Center, Jackson, Mississippi, USA

A. J. Hall MB, BS, LRCP, FRCS
Consultant Orthopaedic Surgeon, Charing Cross Hospital, London;
Regional Adviser in Orthopaedics NW Thames, UK

D. E. Hastings MD, FRCS(C)
The Wellesley Hospital, Toronto, Ontario, Canada

B. Helal MCh(Orth.), FRCS, FRCS(E)
Department of Orthopaedics, The Royal National Orthopaedic
Hospital, The Royal London Hospital and Enfield District Hospital, UK

J. L. Hughes MD
Professor, Department of Orthopedic Surgery, University of
Mississippi Medical Center, Jackson, Mississippi, USA

Cecil H. Rorabeck MD, FRCS(C)
University Hospital, London, Ontario, Canada

John M. Sullivan MB, ChB, FRACS
Department of Orthopaedics, Waikato Hospital, Hamilton, New
Zealand

W. A. Wallace FRCS(Ed), FRCS Ed(Orth)
Professor of Orthopaedic and Accident Surgery, Nottingham
University Hospital, UK

J. K. Webb FRCS
Consultant Orthopaedic Surgeon; Teacher, Spinal Disorders Unit,
Harlow Wood Hospital and Nottingham University Hospital, UK

Contents

Chapter 1

The hip

D. E. Hastings, J. M. Sullivan and C. L. Colton

RELEVANT ANATOMY

Surface anatomy

Bony landmarks readily identified about the hip are as follows: the symphysis pubis, the pubic tubercle, the anterior superior iliac spine, the greater trochanter, the posterior superior iliac spine and the ischial tuberosity. The inguinal ligament runs from the anterior superior iliac spine to the pubic tubercle and corresponds to the groin crease. The mid-point of this line is termed the mid-inguinal point and overlies the femoral head. The sciatic nerve can be located posteriorly at a point midway between the greater trochanter and the ischial tuberosity. The surgical approaches to the hip utilize these landmarks.

Superficial cutaneous nerves

There are two important nerves which have to be considered in choosing the operative incision.

LATERAL FEMORAL CUTANEOUS NERVE OF THE THIGH (Figure 1.1)

This nerve pierces the inguinal ligament 1 cm medial to the anterior superior iliac spine. It crosses sartorius to lie in the interval between sartorius and tensor fascia lata

beneath the deep fascia. Three to four centimetres below the anterior spine, it divides, each branch piercing the deep fascia and supplying skin sensation on the lateral aspect of the thigh from below the greater trochanter to the level of the lateral femoral condyle. This nerve may easily be injured in anterior approaches to the hip.

POSTERIOR CUTANEOUS NERVE OF THE THIGH (Figure 1.2)

This nerve passes through the sciatic notch below piriformis and medial to the sciatic nerve. It then comes to lie between the sciatic nerve and gluteus maximus and continues down the posterior aspect of the thigh almost in the mid-line. It pierces the deep fascia at the level of the gluteal crease and supplies skin sensation from there to below the knee. It is most vulnerable in the low posterior approaches where it lies below the inferior border of gluteus maximus before piercing the deep fascia.

Deep nerves

There are four main nerves which should be considered when planning any approach to the hip.

FEMORAL NERVE (Figure 1.1)

This nerve emerges from the iliac fossa between the iliacus and psoas muscles. It passes deep to the inguinal

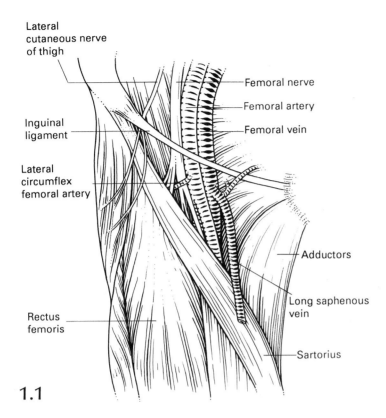

Lateral cutaneous nerve of thigh

Inguinal ligament

Lateral circumflex femoral artery

Rectus femoris

Femoral nerve

Femoral artery

Femoral vein

Adductors

Long saphenous vein

Sartorius

1.1

ligament, just medial to the mid-inguinal point, and lies lateral to the femoral sheath containing the femoral artery and vein. Two or three centimetres below the ligament it divides into muscular and cutaneous branches. The most significant cutaneous branch is the long saphenous nerve which accompanies the saphenous vein distally. The femoral nerve is vulnerable to injury when retractors are placed over the anterior pelvic brim, especially if passed superficial to the psoas muscle. The nerve is also at risk at the time of psoas tenotomy. The muscular branches to vastus lateralis are encountered in an anterolateral approach to the proximal femoral shaft.

SUPERIOR GLUTEAL NERVE (Figure 1.2)

This nerve emerges from the greater sciatic notch above piriformis and crosses the posterior border of gluteus medius with the superior gluteal artery. It then runs anteriorly between gluteus medius and minimus, supplying both, and terminates in the tensor fascia lata, supplying that muscle. It may be injured in the sciatic notch at the time of pelvic osteotomy or posterior column reconstruction after acetabular fracture. It is also vulnerable in a lateral approach when the gluteus medius is split proximally and its terminal branch to tensor fascia lata may be injured in an extensive anterolateral exposure.

OBTURATOR NERVE

This nerve enters the thigh through the obturator notch where it divides into anterior and posterior divisions. The anterior division passes above the obturator externus muscle, continuing into the thigh on the anterior surface of the adductor brevis. The posterior division passes through the upper border of the obturator externus muscle and then continues distally on the adductor magnus.

SCIATIC NERVE (Figure 1.2)

The sciatic nerve emerges from the greater sciatic notch below the piriformis muscle. Initially, it lies on the ischium and then passes, superficial to the obturator internus, gemelli and quadratus femoris, into the posterior compartment of the thigh. It is deep to the gluteus maximus and lies midway between the ischial tuberosity and greater trochanter. This nerve is at risk in trauma to the posterior aspect of the hip, such as posterior dislocation, or posterior column fracture, and may be injured during a posterior approach to the hip joint.

Vessels

LONG SAPHENOUS VEIN (Figure 1.1)

This vein begins on the dorsum of the foot, anterior to the medial malleolus. It runs up the medial aspect of the calf to the knee and becomes anterior in the thigh. It passes through the saphenous opening and femoral sheath to join the femoral vein just below the inguinal ligament. It is joined by a number of large tributaries in the thigh.

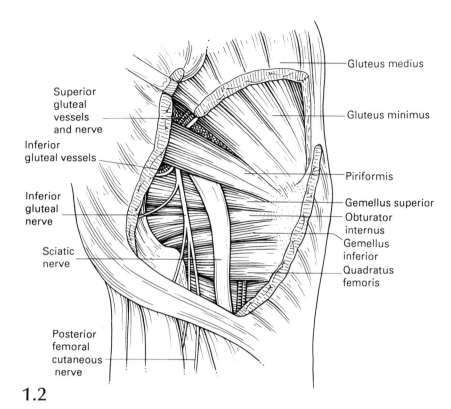

Labels on figure:
- Superior gluteal vessels and nerve
- Inferior gluteal vessels
- Inferior gluteal nerve
- Sciatic nerve
- Posterior femoral cutaneous nerve
- Gluteus medius
- Gluteus minimus
- Piriformis
- Gemellus superior
- Obturator internus
- Gemellus inferior
- Quadratus femoris

1.2

FEMORAL VEIN (Figure 1.1)

This major vessel enters the femoral triangle posterior to the femoral artery and, as it passes upward, it comes to lie medial to the artery. It is joined by the long saphenous vein just inferior to the inguinal ligament and enters the pelvis to become the external iliac vein.

FEMORAL ARTERY (Figure 1.1)

The femoral artery is a continuation of the external iliac artery, and passes beneath the inguinal ligament, inside the femoral sheath. It lies just medial to the mid-inguinal point and leaves the femoral canal deep to sartorius. At the lower border of the femoral sheath, the profunda femoris artery is given off posterolaterally. This passes posteriorly, medially and distally on the anterior surface of iliopsoas and pectineus. After passing anterior to adductor brevis, the profunda femoris artery comes to lie in close proximity to the femur, being separated from the superficial femoral artery by adductor longus. It is in this position that it may be injured by retractors or drills. Aneurysms of this artery have been reported in relation to screws projecting medially beyond the femoral cortex.

MEDIAL CIRCUMFLEX FEMORAL ARTERY

This vessel arises from the medial side of the profunda femoris artery passing between pectineus and psoas. It comes to lie superficial to adductor brevis and at this point passes between adductor magnus and quadratus femoris.

It then sends a horizontal branch along the lower border of quadratus femoris to the cruciate anastomosis and an ascending branch along the upper border of quadratus femoris to the trochanteric anastomosis. These branches form an important source of the blood supply to the femoral head and neck.

LATERAL CIRCUMFLEX FEMORAL ARTERY (Figure 1.1)

This artery may arise from either the lateral side of the profunda femoris artery, or as a direct branch of the femoral artery. It passes between the anterior and posterior divisions of the femoral nerve and leaves the femoral triangle deep to sartorius and rectus femoris. At this point it divides into three branches, the ascending branch to the trochanteric anastomosis, the transverse branch which crosses the vastus lateralis to join the cruciate anastomosis and a descending branch which supplies the vastus lateralis. Major branches of both the medial and lateral circumflex femoral arteries are encountered in exposures of the proximal femoral shaft.

OBTURATOR ARTERY

In company with the obturator nerve, this vessel emerges from the obturator foramen and supplies adjacent muscles. A branch joins the obturator nerve on the anterior surface of adductor brevis and there is a branch that enters the acetabulum deep to the transverse ligament, and may pass to the femoral head via the ligamentum teres.

SUPERIOR GLUTEAL ARTERY (Figure 1.2)

This large vessel is a direct branch of the internal iliac artery. It leaves the pelvis through the greater sciatic notch above piriformis. A superficial branch supplies gluteus maximus and the overlying skin. The deep branch continues laterally in the interval between gluteus medius and minimus accompanying the superior gluteal nerve. This vessel ends by splitting into contributions to the anastomoses at both the anterior superior iliac spine and the greater trochanter. It must be preserved in major myocutaneous flaps during large exposures for fixation of pelvic fractures and it is also vulnerable in the sciatic notch at the time of pelvic osteotomy.

INFERIOR GLUTEAL ARTERY (Figure 1.2)

This vessel is also a branch of the internal iliac artery, exiting from the pelvis through the greater sciatic notch below piriformis. It supplies gluteus maximus and forms an important contribution to the cruciate anastomosis. It can also be injured in osteotomies of the pelvis.

Blood supply to the femoral head and neck

The medial circumflex and lateral circumflex femoral arteries are the predominant stem vessels to the hip joint and its surrounding area. They are joined by a number of vessels to form three important anastomoses. The greatest contribution is from the medial circumflex femoral artery.

The medial circumflex femoral artery, after reaching the back of the femur, supplies an ascending branch which forms the posterior portion of the basal circle. This joins the anterior limb from the lateral circumflex femoral artery and, along with branches from the superior gluteal and superficial circumflex arteries, they form the trochanteric anastomosis. This anastomosis is situated in the region of the trochanteric fossa and gives off branches which pierce the capsule, supply the neck and head, and form the subcapital anastomosis.

The intracapsular arrangement is of two or more arterial systems running in the posterosuperior region of the neck, either in retinacular folds, or actually grooving the femoral neck. A second major intracapsular system arises from the posterior basal circle and runs posteroinferiorly to the femoral neck. An anterior system of less importance is formed from a branch of the lateral circumflex femoral artery.

A branch of the obturator artery enters the acetabulum deep to the transverse acetabular ligament and may pass on to the femoral head through the ligamentum teres. The obturator artery, both gluteal arteries, and the medial circumflex femoral artery also combine to form a third anastomosis, namely the acetabular anastomosis. This supplies surrounding bone, soft tissue and the acetabulum.

In osteoarthritis, osteophyte formation may incorporate the vessels grooving the femoral neck. Furthermore, the direct intramedullary blood supply to the neck and femoral head is increased. These factors play a significant role in vascularization of the femoral head, but cannot guarantee viability if other systems are sacrificed.

Section of the capsule close to the acetabulum provides the best protection for this intricate blood supply. Dissection in the region of the inferior capsule can damage the medial circumflex vessel and a major contribution to the blood supply of the femoral head is lost. The trochanteric anastomosis may be damaged in approaches involving trochanteric osteotomy.

SURGICAL APPROACHES (Figure 1.3)

- Anterior
  Anterior iliofemoral (Smith-Petersen)
  Limited anterior
  Extended ilioinguinal*
- Combined anterior and posterior
  Extended iliofemoral*
  Letournel approach*
  Rüedi approach (see extended transtrochanteric)*
  * For pelvic reconstructions
- Lateral
  Anterolateral (modified Watson-Jones)
  Lateral transgluteal
  Transtrochanteric
  Extended transtrochanteric (Rüedi)
- Posterior
  Posterolateral
  Southern
- Medial
  Medial adductor (Ludloff)

Anterior iliofemoral approach

This is the most commonly used anterior approach. Smith-Petersen (1917) described what is fundamentally the current technique. There are many modifications but, essentially, once beneath the skin the plane to the hip joint is between the tensor fascia lata and sartorius.

Access

This approach allows access to both the inner and outer tables of the ilium, the anterosuperior aspect of the acetabulum, the femoral head and neck and the proximal femoral shaft.

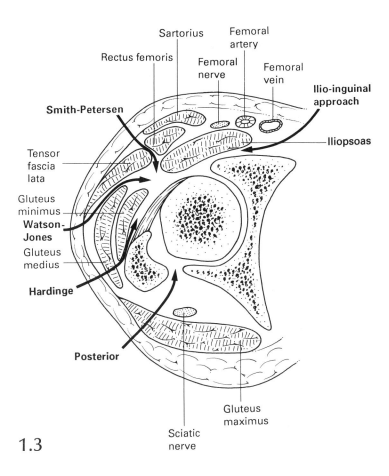

Sartorius

Rectus femoris

Femoral
artery

Femoral
nerve

Femoral
vein

**Ilio-inguinal
approach**

Smith-Petersen

Iliopsoas

Tensor
fascia
lata

Gluteus
minimus

**Watson-
Jones**

Gluteus
medius

Hardinge

Posterior

Gluteus
maximus

Sciatic
nerve

1.3

Position

The patient is placed supine, with the buttock elevated. The leg is draped free, with drapes passing well proximal to the anterior superior iliac spine and posterior to the gluteal tubercle.

Incision (Figure 1.4)

The original Smith-Petersen incision begins at the junction of the middle and anterior thirds of the iliac crest, passes forward to the anterior superior spine and then distally down the thigh over the interval between tensor and sartorius. We prefer an incision in the bikini line parallel to the iliac crest. It begins 4 cm below the mid-portion of the crest, passes forward and distally midway between the anterior superior and anterior inferior iliac spines, terminating at the medial border of sartorius. In children the incision need only be carried 2 cm medial to the anterior superior iliac spine (Somerville, 1953). This produces a cosmetically more acceptable scar.

Approach

Once the deep fascia is encountered, the skin and subcutaneous fat can be mobilized to expose the anterior portion of the iliac crest and proximal anterior thigh (Figure 1.5). An incision is made in the fascia overlying the gluteus medius, just below the iliac crest, extending from the gluteal tubercle to the anterior superior spine. A longitudinal incision is made in the fascia of the anterior thigh over the tensor fascia lata, in order to protect the lateral femoral cutaneous nerve. The interval between tensor fascia lata and sartorius is then deepened to expose a deeper fascial layer. This is opened and the rectus femoris exposed and retracted medially. The ascending branch of the lateral circumflex artery and vein should be identified prior to ligation and division. Dissection is then carried proximally to the anterior inferior iliac spine. The branches of the iliac anastomosis are cauterized as encountered. The capsule of the hip joint can be identified deep to the lateral edge of the rectus femoris. Dividing the reflected head of the rectus will improve the exposure of the superior aspect of the acetabulum. The exposure is then increased by subperiosteal stripping of the muscles off the lateral pelvic wall as far posteriorly as the sciatic notch, if necessary (Figure 1.6). In children, instead of dividing the fascia over the gluteus medius, the cartilaginous apophysis is split longitudinally over the iliac crest, and the subperiosteal dissection is considerably easier.

Improved exposure of the capsule of the hip joint can be obtained by releasing rectus femoris from the anterior inferior iliac spine and by stripping soft tissues off the inferomedial capsule. This exposes the acetabular margin, the superior, anterior and inferior aspects of the hip joint

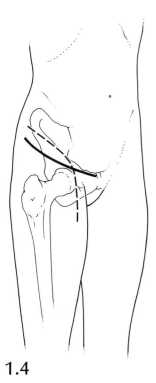

1.4

as far posteriorly as the sacroiliac joint and as far inferiorly as the iliopubic eminence of the superior pubic ramus.

As an alternative to soft tissue release of the abdominal muscles from the iliac crest, an iliac osteotomy, running parallel to the top of the crest and 1 cm distal to it, may be undertaken in its anterior third to anterior half. If this is undertaken carefully and only the outer table and medulla cut with the osteotome, the curved portion of iliac crest can be tilted medially, cracking the inner table of the ilium. This will then permit easy subperiosteal exposure of the inner table down to the greater sciatic notch.

Indications

This approach provides excellent exposure of the acetabulum and anterior pelvic rim. It is an ideal exposure for surgery of congenital dislocation of the hip, where not only can an open reduction be carried out, but it may be combined with pelvic osteotomy. Most types of pelvic

capsule and the lesser trochanter. The capsule can be incised along the acetabular margin and a 'T' incision made down to the anterior femoral neck allowing wide exposure (Figure 1.7). Dislocation of the femoral head may be accomplished by external rotation and adduction.

If further relaxation and exposure are required, the incision may be extended more posteriorly on the iliac crest stripping gluteus medius from the lateral pelvic wall. Moreover, the inguinal ligament may be released, and by release of the attachment of the abdominal muscles, subperiosteal exposure of the inner table can be extended

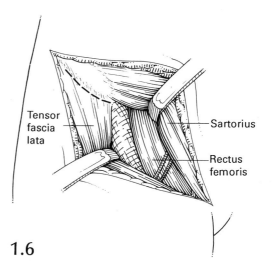

1.6

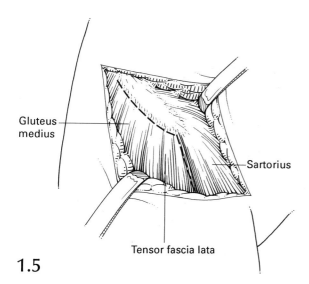

1.5

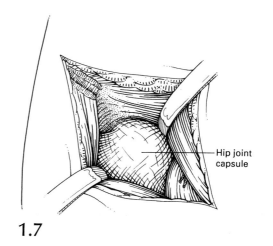

1.7

osteotomy are best done by this approach. It would be the approach of choice for traumatic anterior dislocation, as well as for the reduction of major fractures of the upper portion of the anterior column or of the iliac wing.

Advantages

1. Excellent acetabular exposure allowing major reconstruction.
2. Ready source of bone graft material.
3. Relaxation of gluteal muscles in cases of high-riding dislocations.
4. Preservation of blood supply of femoral head by posterior retinacular vessels.
5. Extensile to proximal femoral shaft.

Disadvantages

1. Major muscle dissection results in the necessity for prolonged protection to avoid the risk of late detachment of the tensor fascia lata and gluteus medius.
2. The incidence of heterotopic bone formation and subsequent joint stiffness is higher.
3. Injury to the lateral femoral cutaneous nerve, with disturbing dysaesthesia of the thigh, is a common problem.
4. Exposure of the femoral medullary canal is limited.
5. Moderate incisional pain, if the abdominal muscles are released.

Limited anterior approach

This approach is essentially the distal part of the anterior iliofemoral exposure. This approach utilizes the interval between tensor fascia lata and sartorius, without detaching either the tensor or glutei from the outer table of the ilium.

Access

Limited direct anterior access to hip joint.

Position

The patient is supine with buttock elevated and the leg draped free.

Incision

A short oblique incision is made 4 cm below the anterior superior iliac spine (Figure 1.8).

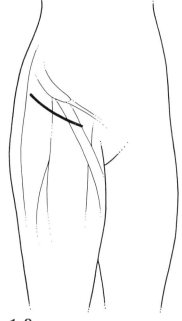

1.8

Approach

The skin and subcutaneous tissues are elevated proximally and distally to expose the deep fascia. The fascia lata is divided longitudinally to develop the interval between tensor fascia lata and sartorius. Dissection then proceeds along the lateral border of rectus femoris, dividing the deep fascia (Figure 1.9). Branches of the lateral circumflex artery and vein are ligated and divided. The rectus femoris is elevated to expose the anterior capsule of the hip joint and released if more exposure is required. The iliopsoas tendon and lesser trochanter can also be reached through this approach.

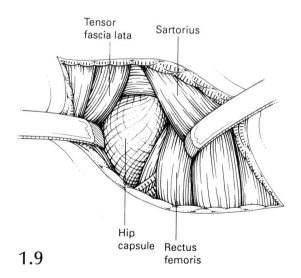

Tensor fascia lata   Sartorius

Hip capsule   Rectus femoris

1.9

Indications

This approach allows exposure of the anterior hip capsule without detachment of the hip abductors, and therefore has a reduced morbidity. It is suitable for biopsy of the synovium and femoral head, drainage of septic arthritis, and soft tissue releases, such as anterior capsulotomy and psoas tenotomy.

Advantages

1. Cosmetic, relatively small skin incision.
2. Reduced morbidity because of preservation of gluteal origin.
3. Extensile to iliofemoral approach.

Disadvantages

1. Risk of injury to lateral femoral cutaneous nerve.
2. Limited exposure.

Ilioinguinal approach

This approach was originally described by the Judet brothers and Letournel in 1964 for wide access to fractures of the acetabulum, particularly involving the anterior column.

Access

In the extended form it will give access to the interior of the hemi-pelvis over an area bounded by the ala of the sacrum posteriorly, the iliac crest superiorly, the sciatic notch inferomedially and the symphysis pubis anteriorly.

Position

The patient is placed supine, with the ipsilateral buttock elevated and the leg draped free. The drapes must allow access posteriorly to the anterior three-quarters of the iliac crest and to the mid-line anteriorly.

Incision

Starting at the junction of the posterior and middle thirds of the iliac crest, a bikini-type incision is made, extending to the mid-line at the superior border of the symphysis pubis. This incision curves convex distally (Figure 1.10). The skin and subcutaneous fat are elevated to expose the iliac crest and, from the anterior superior iliac spine to the mid-line, to expose the inguinal ligament and the external abdominal muscles which form the anterior wall of the inguinal canal.

Approach

There are two variants of this approach; the original described by Judet *et al.* passes above the inguinal ligament and through the inguinal canal. The variation described by Rüedi detaches the anterior superior iliac spine with the outer attachment of the inguinal ligament and, elevating this, together with the attached abdominal muscles, allows an approach inferior to the inguinal ligament.

Judet and Letournel approach

In the iliac region, either the abdominal muscles are detached from the iliac crest by soft tissue incision, or the anterior one-third to one-half of the iliac crest is osteotomized, raising a curved, crest fragment, the inner table of which is fractured by tilting the fragment medially, permitting subperiosteal dissection inside the iliac wing. The abdominal muscles are released from the junction of the posterior and middle thirds of the iliac crest to the anterior superior iliac spine. Subperiosteal detachment of the iliacus muscle from the inner table of the wing of the ilium is then undertaken as far posteriorly as the sacroiliac joint, if necessary. In the abdominal extent of the incision, the aponeurosis of the external oblique muscle is divided from the anterior superior iliac spine to the mid-line, taking particular care not only to avoid damage to the lateral cutaneous nerve of the thigh just medial to the anterior superior iliac spine, but also to carry the incision of the aponeurosis *above* the external inguinal orifice (Figure 1.11). The conjoint tendon and its attachment to the inguinal ligament are thereby exposed. Sharp dissection of this tendon from the inguinal ligament through the tendinous fibres of origin is then undertaken, leaving a tough fibrous strip which assists in reattachment during closure. This exposes the iliopsoas muscle mass with the femoral nerve lying on its anterior surface, the abdominal muscles being retracted upwards. The fascia overlying the iliopsoas muscle mass is carefully divided and at the medial border of the muscle mass this fascia merges with

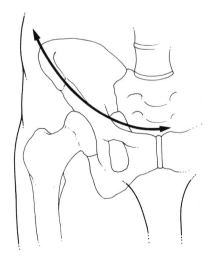

1.10

the iliopectineal band, which should also be divided at its attachment to the pelvic bone (Figure 1.12(a)). The iliopsoas muscle mass, together with the femoral nerve, can then be isolated and a length of latex tubing passed around it to permit its retraction in either direction. Medial to the iliopsoas muscle mass lies the femoral sheath, containing the femoral artery and the femoral vein. This needs to be dissected carefully and a piece of latex tubing passed around the sheath to permit its retraction in either direction. Medial to the femoral sheath in the male lies the spermatic cord which should also be mobilized, isolated and retracted using latex tubing. This then gives three soft tissue bundles; laterally the iliopsoas muscle mass, in the centre the femoral sheath and vessels and medially the spermatic cord (Figure 1.12(b)). Deep to these three soft tissue bundles lies the superior pubic ramus which can be exposed throughout the whole of its

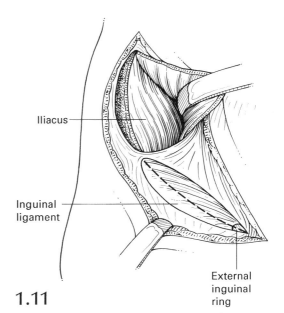

1.11

length, section by section, by retracting the appropriate soft tissue bundle(s) in either direction. If a more medial extension of the approach is required then the tendinous attachments to the pectineal line and to the superior portion of the body of the pubis will need to be incised, leaving a sufficient cuff of tissue to permit subsequent repair (Figure 1.12(c)). If necessary, the incision can be carried across the mid-line to expose the contralateral pubis, even combining bilateral ilioinguinal approaches for exposure of the whole anterior brim of the pelvis in complex pelvic injuries.

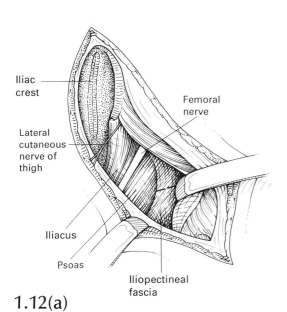

1.12(a)

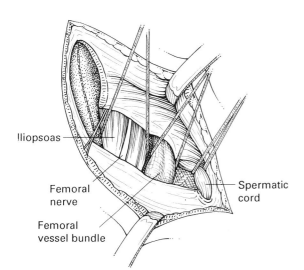

1.12(b)

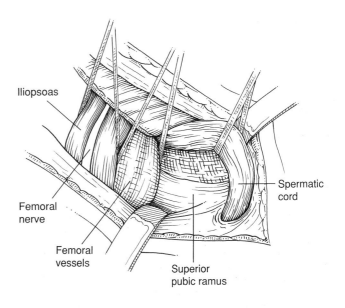

1.12(c)

Warning. An anatomical variant of the vascular anatomy in this region is a large vessel bridging between the inferior epigastric artery and the obturator artery – the so-called 'corona mortis' passing behind the body of the pubis. Inadvertent damage to this vessel should be avoided, lest troublesome haemorrhage result.

Rüedi approach

This approach is similar in principle to the Judet and Letournel approach, but passes inferior to the inguinal ligament which is detached from the pelvis laterally by osteotomy of the anterior superior iliac spine. The iliac extent of this approach is accomplished as above, preferably with osteotomy of the anterior half of the iliac crest, including the anterior superior iliac spine. In the anterior portion of the approach, the fascia along the inferior border of the inguinal ligament is incised and the bone fragment from the iliac crest, including the anterior superior iliac spine, together with the inguinal ligament and the external abdominal muscles, are retracted superiorly and medially (Figure 1.13). It is at this point that the lateral cutaneous nerve of the thigh should be sought and if possible preserved. The inguinal ligament is then elevated as far as its insertion at the pubic tubercle. The exposure and mobilization of the iliopsoas muscle mass, together with the femoral nerve on its anterior surface and also of the femoral sheath, are as described above. Any extension of the approach medial to the femoral sheath involves the passage of a latex tube around the spermatic cord where it emerges from the external inguinal orifice and then, medial to this, transverse division of the muscular attachments to the medial end of the superior pubic ramus and the superior portion of the body of the pubis, leaving a sufficient cuff of tissue for subsequent repair. This approach can be combined with a similar approach on the contralateral side for exposure of the whole anterior brim of the pelvis in complex pelvic fractures.

Closure

Any division of the rectus abdominis muscles must be repaired at their attachment to the pubis and the anterior rectus sheath sutured. In the Judet and Letournel approach the conjoint tendon of origin from the inguinal ligament is carefully repaired and the external abdominal muscles are repaired and reattached to the iliac crest using sutures anchored, if necessary, in the fascia covering the gluteus medius muscle. The skin and fat are then closed. One or more vacuum drains are normally used.

In the Rüedi approach, the repair of the muscles arising from the superior portion of the body of the pubis and the medial end of the superior pubic ramus is undertaken, the bony fragment of anterior crest and anterior superior iliac spine is reattached, using lag screws, and any soft tissue division of the anterior abdominal muscles from the iliac crest is repaired. The skin and fat are then closed; one or more vacuum drains are used.

Indications

As discussed above, this approach affords very wide access to the inner side of the hemi-pelvis and to the anterior column of the acetabulum. The anterior aspect of the sacroiliac joint may be exposed, permitting anterior osteosynthesis of dislocations and subluxations of the sacroiliac joint. It does not permit exposure for internal fixation of fractures through the ala of the sacrum, and great care must be taken in the posterior reaches of this

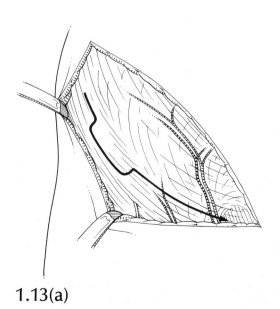

1.13(a)

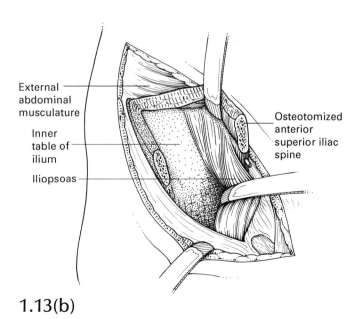

External abdominal musculature

Inner table of ilium

Iliopsoas

Osteotomized anterior superior iliac spine

1.13(b)

incision, the dissection sticking closely to bone throughout. Transverse and anterior column fractures of the acetabulum are admirably dealt with through this approach. On the inner aspect of the pelvis extension of the field of view down to the greater sciatic notch will permit reduction and lag screw fixation of the posterior column in some transverse fractures. This, however, requires considerable surgical experience. Fractures of the anterior column, the superior pubic ramus and even disruptions of the pubic symphysis will be dealt with by this approach, if necessary in combination with a limited contralateral anterior ilioinguinal exposure.

Advantages

1. Wide field of exposure for complex pelvic fractures, particularly the anterior column distal to the iliopubic eminence.
2. Cosmetically acceptable scar, provided skin suture is fine, gentle and meticulous.
3. Less tendency to heterotopic ossification

Disadvantages

1. Possible damage to the lateral cutaneous nerve of the thigh.
2. Possible damage to the 'corona mortis'.
3. Possible damage to the external iliac and femoral vessels. Their careful liberation by blunt dissection using the finger not only avoids this but avoids damage to the lymphatics which accompany them.
4. This approach requires great surgical expertise and patient, meticulous, surgical technique with a detailed knowledge of anatomy. It is strongly recommended that even the experienced surgeon practise this approach in the post-mortem room before attempting it either for the first time or for the first time after a long interval.

Extended iliofemoral approach of Judet and Letournel

In 1964 the brothers Judet and Letournel described this approach which offers an extensive exposure of the hemi-pelvis for the management of complex fractures of the acetabulum.

Access

Access is gained to the whole of the posterior column of the acetabulum, the superior or dome portion and the anterior column as far distally as the iliopubic eminence.

Position

The patient is placed in the lateral decubitus position and held stable in this position with appropriate attachments to the operating table. A distal femoral transcondylar skeletal traction pin should be inserted and a stirrup then attached to permit traction along the femur in the surgical management of acetabular fractures. The knee should be kept flexed to a right angle at all times to provide relaxation of the sciatic nerve.

Incision

The incision parallels the anterior three-quarters of the iliac crest as far as the anterior superior iliac spine and then curves distally following a line joining the anterior superior iliac spine and the lateral border of the patella. The incision usually extends to the mid-thigh (Figure 1.14).

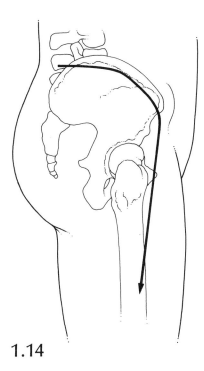

1.14

Approach

The interval between the sartorius and tensor fascia lata muscles is developed and the division of the deep fascia is continued distally in the line of the skin incision to expose the outer surface of the greater trochanter and the lateral surface of vastus lateralis. At this stage the tendinous insertions of the gluteus medius and minimus muscles into the greater trochanter are divided 1–2 cm from their insertion, leaving sufficient tendon tissue to permit later resuture. The alternative of trochanteric osteotomy is discussed in the Rüedi approach (see page 17).

The next stage is the subperiosteal detachment of the gluteus medius and minimus from the outer surface of the

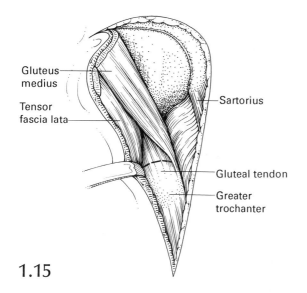

Gluteus medius

Tensor fascia lata

Sartorius

Gluteal tendon

Greater trochanter

1.15

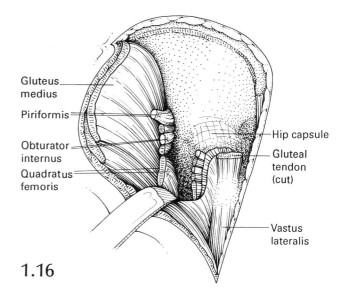

Gluteus medius

Piriformis

Obturator internus

Quadratus femoris

Hip capsule

Gluteal tendon (cut)

Vastus lateralis

1.16

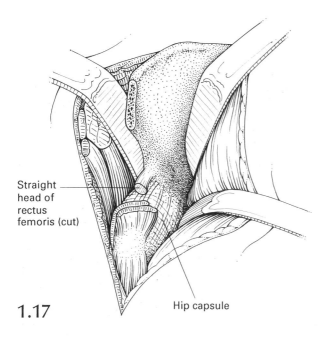

Straight head of rectus femoris (cut)

Hip capsule

1.17

wing of the ilium as already described for the standard iliofemoral approach. This dissection is carried back to the greater sciatic notch. This permits retraction of the whole muscle mass of the gluteus medius and minimus as far back as the greater sciatic notch (Figure 1.15). Great care must be taken to preserve the superior gluteal neurovascular bundle as this is now the sole 'life-line' to the muscle mass. In the retraction of the mass, these vessels must not be kinked or obstructed in any way. Frequently during the progress of the operation this muscle mass should gently be replaced, covered by moist towels and a short break taken to permit full perfusion of the muscular tissue.

The external rotator muscles are detached from their insertion to the posterior edge of the greater trochanter starting superiorly with piriformis, and continuing distally through the gemellus superior, obturator internus, gemellus inferior and quadratus femoris. Stay sutures in these tendons permit their retraction posteriorly, thereby protecting the sciatic nerve. Periosteal dissection deep to these muscles exposes the posterior column of the acetabulum (Figure 1.16). At the point where the tendon of obturator internus loops round the sciatic notch, deep to the short external rotator muscles, there is a small bursa directly on the bone of the notch and this affords a safe site for the careful insertion of a pointed lever retractor of the Hohman type.

The next stage is to divide the straight and reflected heads of rectus femoris, allowing this muscle to be retracted medially. The abdominal muscles are then divided from the iliac crest (or a crest osteotomy performed, as described above), permitting the subperiosteal elevation of the iliacus muscle from the inner table of the pelvis. At the anterior brim of the pelvis, level with the hip joint, periosteal dissection can continue along the anterior column of the hip, as far distally as the iliopubic eminence with medial retraction of the muscle mass composed of the iliacus muscle, the psoas muscle and the rectus femoris. Flexion of the hip at this stage relaxes these anterior structures (Figure 1.17).

Closure

This consists of reattachment of the abdominal muscles (combined with internal fixation of the curved iliac crest fragment, if this has been elevated), resuture of the fascia overlying the gluteus medius and minimus muscles at the iliac crest and careful resuture, using non-absorbable material, of the tendons of insertion of the gluteus medius and minimus into the greater trochanter. Stay sutures previously placed in the two cut ends of the tendons of each of piriformis and obturator internus can then be used to reattach these muscles. Multiple vacuum drains are normally used.

Advantages

1. A large exposure of the hemi-pelvis for the majority of acetabular fractures, particularly those involving both anterior and posterior columns.

Disadvantages

1. Exposure of the anterior column limited to its superior portion.
2. Division of the tendons of gluteus medius and minimus necessitates a more prolonged period of protected weight-bearing.

Note

A variant of this approach, detaching the tip of the greater trochanter rather than dividing the tendons of insertion of gluteus medius and minimus, has been devised by Rüedi (1984) and is described later as the extended trans-trochanteric approach.

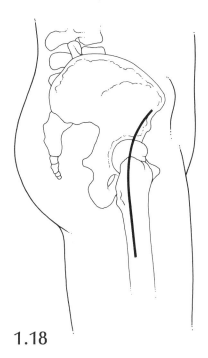

1.18

Anterolateral approach (modified Watson-Jones)

Ollier in 1881 first described the lateral approach to the hip by a U-shaped incision. Other authors modified the approach and Watson-Jones (1936) described the current approach. Müller adapted and popularized this approach for performing his total hip replacement procedure.

Access

This approach gives access to the anterior capsule of the hip joint, acetabulum, lateral pelvic wall and proximal femur.

Position

The patient is supine with two small rolled towels under each buttock. This keeps the patient level and allows the soft tissues to fall away from the trochanter. The leg is draped free.

Incision

The incision begins 2 cm posterior to the anterior superior iliac spine, curves distally and posteriorly to the greater trochanter and then passes down the thigh for 5 cm (Figure 1.18).

Approach

The fascia lata is identified and incised along the posterior border of the greater trochanter. Distally, the fascia is split longitudinally, the cut curving slightly, concave anteriorly. Proximally, the fascial incision is curved up to the anterior superior iliac spine. The adipose tissue is cleaned off the vastus lateralis and this introduces the surgeon to the interval between gluteus medius and tensor fascia lata (Figure 1.19). This interval is developed proximally for 5–6 cm. Small vessels are cauterized as encountered. Care must be taken to avoid dissecting too proximally where there is a risk of injuring the terminal branch of the superior gluteal nerve to the tensor fascia lata.

The gluteus minimus tendon is isolated and divided and the anterior part of the insertion of gluteus medius into the greater trochanter is also released. This exposes the superior capsule. The rectus femoris is then elevated and a retractor placed deep to it, over the pelvic brim to expose the anterior capsule. Finally, the inferior aspect of the capsule is cleared and a retractor placed deep to the psoas tendon and against the inferior acetabular margin, to provide a wide exposure of the hip capsule (Figure 1.20). The capsule may then be incised or excised. It can be difficult to dislocate the femoral head through this exposure, and in arthroplasty transection of the femoral neck prior to removal of the head is often advisable. Exposure of the acetabulum is facilitated by division of the posterior capsule and posterior retraction of the femoral neck.

Indications

This approach has been used for total hip arthroplasty. It is a good approach to the femoral head and neck. It is the approach of choice for open reduction of displaced

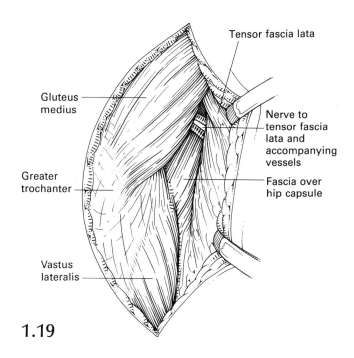

Tensor fascia lata

Gluteus medius

Nerve to tensor fascia lata and accompanying vessels

Greater trochanter

Fascia over hip capsule

Vastus lateralis

1.19

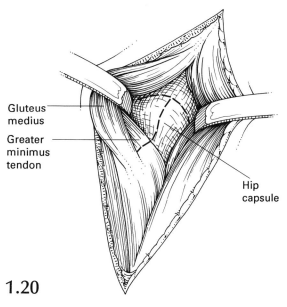

Gluteus medius

Greater minimus tendon

Hip capsule

1.20

intracapsular fractures of the femoral neck and is a suitable approach for capsular release combined with psoas tenotomy. It is not recommended for revision arthroplasty.

Advantages

1. Gluteal origin preserved.
2. Rapid rehabilitation and resumption of weight bearing.

Disadvantages

1. Relatively poor exposure of femoral neck.
2. Risk of damage to gluteus medius and minimus.

Lateral approaches

Two lateral approaches are currently recommended for consideration; the transgluteal and transtrochanteric. McFarland and Osborne (1954) described an approach in which the gluteus medius was split proximally and the incision was carried down into the vastus lateralis, stripping both the gluteus medius and vastus lateralis anteriorly as a single tissue layer, in direct functional continuity. We have termed this the transgluteal approach. Hardinge (1982) described a modification of this approach for total hip replacement.

The transtrochanteric approach was described initially by Ollier in 1881, and then by Brackett in 1912.

Watson-Jones also described trochanteric osteotomy in 1936. It was Sir John Charnley, however, who refined and popularized this approach in his development of the total hip arthroplasty.

TRANSGLUTEAL APPROACH (HARDINGE)

Access

This approach provides good exposure of both the acetabulum and the proximal femur.

Position

The patient may be in the lateral position or in the supine position with the ipsilateral buttock elevated. In either case, the leg is draped free.

Incision

A midlateral incision is made centred over the greater trochanter and extending from the level of the anterior superior iliac spine to a point 6 cm below the greater trochanter (Figure 1.21).

Approach

The fascia lata is incised along the posterior margin of the greater trochanter and continued proximally and distally in the line of the skin incision. The gluteus medius and its insertion into the greater trochanter are identified. This is

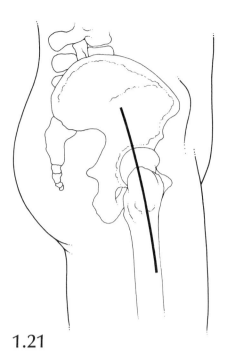

1.21

attachment of gluteus medius to the trochanter, together with the attached periosteum and fascia of the vastus lateralis, is then lifted as a single layer from the anterior portion of the trochanter using a sharp chisel (Figure 1.22). The combined muscle mass is displaced forward. The tendon of gluteus minimus is then divided and the capsule of the hip joint exposed. Two areas of bleeding may be encountered, one from the ascending branch of the medial circumflex femoral artery behind the greater trochanter and the second from the transverse branch of the lateral circumflex femoral artery deep to the vastus lateralis. These are cauterized. After exposure of the anterior capsule (Figure 1.23) a retractor is placed over the pelvic brim, deep to the rectus femoris and directly on bone. The capsule is then incised longitudinally and dissected off the acetabular margin. With a generous capsular incision it is possible to dislocate the hip anteriorly with relative ease (Figure 1.24). After removal of the femoral head and neck excellent exposure of the acetabulum is obtained. In the supine position, the exposure of the femoral neck and medullary cavity is also satisfactory.

If the patient is positioned laterally, the draping should be such that the foot can be placed into a sterile envelope. Lateral positioning allows the possibility of posterior capsulotomy and posterior dislocation of the femoral head. Visualization of the femoral shaft is better and the lateral position is recommended for revision surgery.

facilitated by internal rotation of the hip. The muscle is split in the direction of its fibres at the junction of the anterior and middle thirds. This split is carried proximally 4 cm from the posterosuperior tip of the greater trochanter. An incision is then made down to bone over the trochanter, carried slightly anteriorly and then continued distally into the vastus lateralis along the anterolateral surface of the femur, for a distance of 5 cm. The

Closure

The incision is closed in layers. The gluteus medius, in continuity with vastus lateralis, tends to fall back into the anatomical position and is fixed with interrupted sutures to the remaining posterior musculotendinous tissues. The fascia lata is then closed.

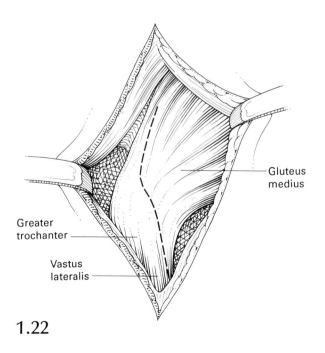

Greater trochanter

Vastus lateralis

Gluteus medius

1.22

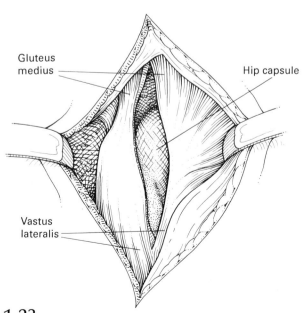

Gluteus medius

Hip capsule

Vastus lateralis

1.23

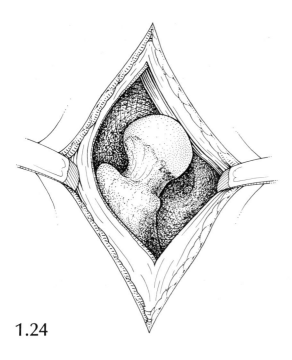

1.24

Indications

This is a very good approach for femoral head or total hip replacement, providing good exposure of both acetabulum and femur. In the lateral position it is an excellent approach for revision of total hip replacement.

Advantages

1. Improved exposure of acetabulum and femoral neck.
2. Greater trochanter preserved, allowing rapid rehabilitation.

Disadvantages

1. Slight increase in blood loss compared with the anterolateral approach.
2. Risk of gluteal weakness, particularly in revision surgery.

Transtrochanteric approach

Access

A very wide exposure of the hip is obtained on both the acetabular and femoral sides.

Position

The patient is usually positioned supine but can be in the lateral position. The leg is draped free.

Incision

A straight lateral incision is made, centred over the greater trochanter, extending proximally 5–6 cm to the level of the anterior superior iliac spine and distally 6–8 cm (Figure 1.25).

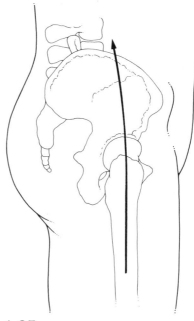

1.25

Approach

The fascia lata is divided in line with the skin incision, towards the posterior aspect of the greater trochanter, and the rough line is identified. Dissection is carried out in the interval between tensor fascia lata and gluteus medius to expose the anterior capsule of the hip joint, similar to the plane described in the anterolateral approach. The posterior margin of gluteus medius is then identified. A curved forceps is introduced directly on the capsule, passing from the anterior edge of gluteus medius to its posterior margin. Abduction and internal rotation of the leg facilitates passage of this forceps. The origin of vastus lateralis is reflected distally from the rough line for a short distance (Figure 1.26). An osteotomy of the greater trochanter is performed from just below the rough line inferiorly, passing up to the curved forceps at the junction of the trochanter and the superior neck. This may be done with an osteotome or can be made from proximal to distal with a Gigli saw. Care must be taken that the osteotomy includes the posterior margin of the greater trochanter. The trochanter with the attached glutei is then freed of

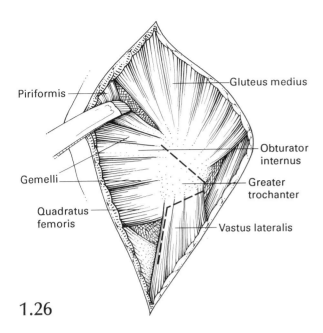

Piriformis

Gluteus medius

Obturator
internus

Gemelli

Greater
trochanter

Quadratus
femoris

Vastus lateralis

1.26

capsular attachments and retracted proximally, after
dividing the tendon of piriformis (Figure 1.27). The
anterior capsule is next exposed by retracting the rectus
femoris medially. The capsule may be opened in a 'T'
fashion, or excised widely. In either case, dislocation by
external rotation, flexion and adduction is relatively easy.

A smaller trochanteric osteotomy may be desirable in

Osteotomized
greater
trochanter

Piriformis

Ilium

Glutei

Hip capsule

Sciatic
nerve

Vastus lateralis

1.27

revision of a total hip replacement. Müller has described a
modification where the trochanter is cut in a chevron
fashion. This is said to provide rotational control,
improved fixation, and more predictable trochanteric
union. The trochanter may be reattached by a tension
band wiring technique or by the use of lag screws.

Indications

Many surgeons still use this as their standard approach for
total hip replacement. It gives the best exposure and is
often indicated in difficult primary reconstructions or for
revisions.

Advantages

1. Wide exposure of acetabulum, femoral neck and canal.
2. Gluteus medius and minimus not damaged.
3. Trochanter may be advanced to improve stability.

Disadvantages

1. Blood loss is increased.
2. Requires longer protection from full load bearing.
3. Delayed or non-union of the trochanter is a significant
   problem in many series.
4. Trochanteric bursitis may be a problem.

Extended transtrochanteric approach

This is an adaptation of other transtrochanteric
approaches such as those of Charnley and Senegas,
described by Rüedi (1984). It is particularly designed for
the management of complex acetabular fractures. It is
analgous to the extended iliofemoral approach of Judet
and Letournel previously described.

Access

This approach gives excellent access to the posterior
column of the acetabulum down as far as the ischial
tuberosity, the superior acetabular dome and the superior
portion of the anterior column of the acetabulum as far
distally as the iliopubic eminence.

Position

A lateral decubitus position is used, the patient being
stabilized either with attachments to the operating table,
or with the use of a vacuum mattress. The limb is draped
free and the operation area draped to expose the

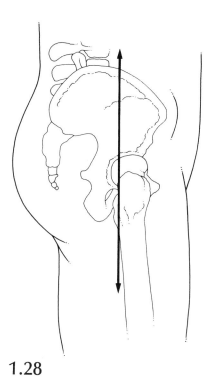

1.28

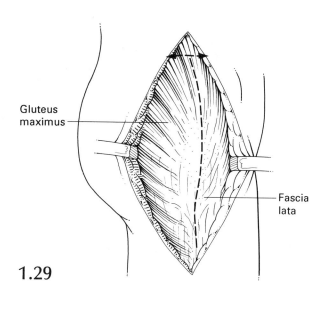

1.29

gluteus maximus muscle, on the deep surface of which are found the superficial branches of the superior gluteal vessels and also the inferior gluteal vessels. The iliotibial tract is detached from the superficial surface of gluteus medius by sharp dissection. The anterior and posterior borders of gluteus medius are exposed, as are the superficial surfaces of the short external rotator muscles of the hip joint and the outer surface of vastus lateralis (Figure 1.30). An extracapsular osteotomy of the greater trochanter is performed and this permits sub-periosteal elevation of the gluteus medius and minimus, superiorly

symphysis pubis anteriorly, the lateral half of the buttock posteriorly, the costal margin proximally and the mid-thigh distally. A distal femoral skeletal traction pin should be inserted and fitted with a stirrup to permit traction along the limb during the reduction of acetabular fractures. The knee should be kept flexed at all times to relax the sciatic nerve.

Incision

A straight lateral incision starts just above the iliac crest and is carried along a line which passes over the posterior edge of the greater trochanter and then extends into the thigh along a line joining the tip of the greater trochanter to the outer border of the patella. The incision is usually carried 10–15 cm below the greater trochanter (Figure 1.28).

Approach

The skin and subcutaneous fat are dissected from the deep fascia, more widely proximally than distally. The deep fascia is divided in the line of the skin incision from distal to proximal. This divides the fascia lata distally and, proximally, the fascia covering gluteus medius as far as the iliac crest.

The incision may then be continued proximally in a 'T' fashion by dividing the iliotibial tract anteriorly and posteriorly, parallel to, and slightly distal to, the iliac crest (Figure 1.29). The flaps of deep fascia are then raised from the underlying muscles, the posterior flap including the

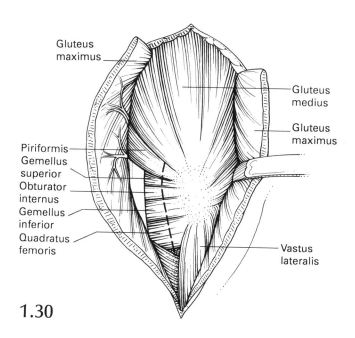

1.30

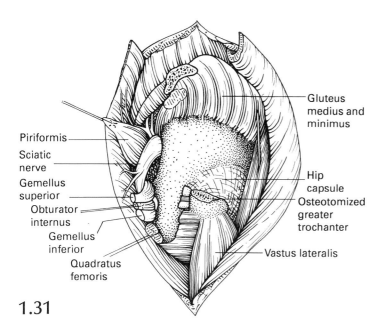

Piriformis

Sciatic
nerve

Gemellus
superior

Obturator
internus

Gemellus
inferior

Quadratus
femoris

Gluteus
medius and
minimus

Hip
capsule

Osteotomized
greater
trochanter

Vastus lateralis

1.31

and posteriorly as far as the greater sciatic notch (Figure 1.31). Great care must be taken of the superior gluteal neurovascular pedicle as it is the only remaining blood supply to the whole muscle mass. Throughout the procedure this muscle mass should be replaced at frequent intervals for several minutes to allow full perfusion. Extreme care must be taken with any retractors used in the region of the superior portion of the greater sciatic notch.

The tendons of piriformis, gemellus superior, obturator internus, gemellus inferior and quadratus femoris are then divided near their insertion into the posterior border of the greater trochanter. Stay sutures in the cut ends of the piriformis and obturator internus tendons permit their posterior retraction to protect the sciatic nerve and also assist in their reinsertion during closure. During division of the quadratus femoris the deep branch of the medial circumflex femoral artery will need to be secured and ligated. Access to the anterior column is gained by division of the straight and reflected heads of rectus femoris. Flexion of the hip will then allow medial retraction of the tensor fascia lata and the iliopsoas muscle as it crosses the anterior pelvic brim. Further access may be gained by osteotomizing the iliac crest, or detaching the abdominal muscles, to permit subperiosteal dissection of the iliacus muscle from the inner table of the ilium. This permits palpation of the inner aspect of the acetabulum to check reduction of fragments and also to permit more accurate directional guidance of drills.

Closure

The osteotomized iliac crest is reattached using lag screws. The tendons of piriformis and obturator internus are reattached to the posterior rim of the greater trochanter using the previously placed stay sutures. The greater trochanteric osteotomy is then repaired using lag

screws or a tension band wiring technique. The iliotibial tract is repaired and the skin and subcutaneous tissue closed. Multiple vacuum drains are normally used.

Posterior approaches

Von Langenbeck (1874) and Kocher (1887) were the first to describe this approach. Many modifications have been made over the subsequent years. In 1945, Henry renewed interest, and, in 1950, Alexander Gibson described a variation of the approach that lead to its resurgence. Moore (1957) described his 'Southern' version for insertion of his femoral head replacement arthroplasty. A universal posterolateral approach is described below.

POSTEROLATERAL

Access

This approach gives good exposure of the posterior lip of the acetabulum and its posterior column, the acetabulum itself, and of the proximal femur, including the femoral medullary canal.

Position

The patient is placed in the lateral position, supported by kidney rests, or by chest and lumbar supports. The leg is draped free. The knee is flexed and kept flexed throughout the procedure to reduce tension on the sciatic nerve.

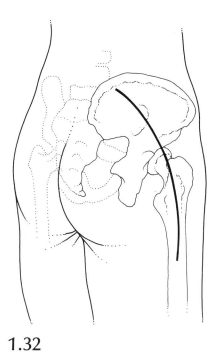

1.32

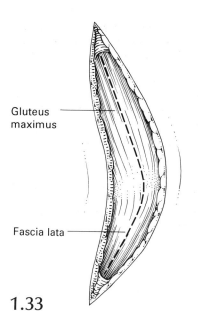

Gluteus maximus

Fascia lata

1.33

Incision

The incision is centred posterior to the prominence of the greater trochanter extending distally 8–10 cm along the lateral thigh. Proximally it is curved gently posteriorly approximately 8 cm towards a point 4 cm anterior to the posterior superior iliac spine (Figure 1.32).

Approach

The fascia lata is incised over the trochanter and split distally in the line of the skin incision. Proximally, the fibres of gluteus maximus are split by blunt dissection, the posterior flap containing almost the entire muscle (Figures 1.33, 1.34). Retracting this posterior flap and with further blunt dissection the sciatic nerve is identifiable in the depths of the incision. The fatty areolar tissue overlying the short external rotators is cleared by blunt dissection.

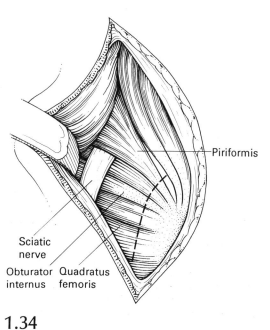

Piriformis

Sciatic nerve

Obturator internus   Quadratus femoris

1.34

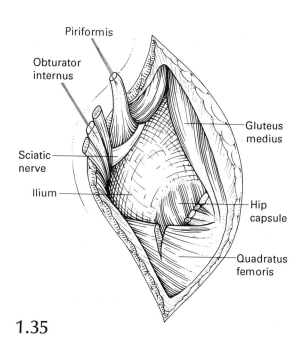

Piriformis

Obturator internus

Sciatic nerve

Ilium

Gluteus medius

Hip capsule

Quadratus femoris

1.35

This is facilitated by gentle internal rotation of the hip (Figure 1.34). Stay sutures are placed through the tendons of piriformis and obturator internus and the short external rotators are divided close to their trochanteric insertions. While retracted posteriorly they serve as a soft tissue protection for the sciatic nerve (Figure 1.35). The quadratus femoris can be divided in part or in whole depending on the required exposure. At its superior border, branches of the medial circumflex femoral artery will need to be identified and ligated. Further exposure can be achieved by division of the gluteus maximus insertion into the femur.

The capsule is incised posteriorly along the femoral neck.

It may be preserved or resected. The hip may be dislocated by flexion, adduction and internal rotation. This should be performed gently to avoid fracture of the femoral neck or shaft, particularly in the osteoporotic elderly patient.

Increased exposure of the superior and anterior aspects of the acetabulum can be achieved by trochanteric osteotomy.

Indications

This approach was widely used for unipolar femoral head replacement in displaced subcapital fractures, although the Hardinge transgluteal approach carries less risk of infection and/or dislocation. It may also be used for primary total joint replacement and revision of a loose femoral component. It is the approach of choice for open reduction of posterior dislocations of the hip, particularly with fractures of the posterior acetabular margin or posterior column. It is a useful approach for exploration of the sciatic nerve. It was originally described for drainage of septic arthritis of the hip.

Advantages

1. Familiar quick approach allowing excellent visualization of the femoral neck and femoral medullary canal.
2. Bleeding is minimized in this approach.

Disadvantages

1. Incision is dependent and subject to oedema.
2. There is an increased incidence of posterior dislocation and of infection following hip arthroplasty.

Southern approach (Moore)

Access

This approach gives access to the proximal sciatic nerve, the posterior and superior aspects of the hip joint and to the femoral neck.

Position

The patient is placed in the lateral position or semi-prone. The affected extremity is draped free.

Incision

The incision begins 10 cm distal to the posterior superior iliac spine, extends laterally to the greater trochanter and then distally along the lateral thigh (Figure 1.36).

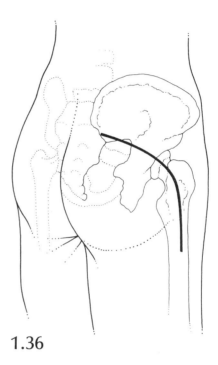

1.36

Approach

The fascia lata is divided over the greater trochanter and continued proximally and distally in the line of the skin incision. The fibres of gluteus maximus are separated by blunt dissection, care being taken to avoid disturbing the inferior gluteal vessels in the most proximal corner of the exposure. The gluteus maximus is retracted posteriorly and its tendinous insertion into the linea aspera divided, if necessary. This provides good exposure of the sciatic nerve which is retracted with care. The dissection then proceeds in an identical fashion to that described in the posterolateral exposure. The piriformis, the obturator internus and the gemelli are cleared and divided at their trochanteric insertions (Figure 1.35). The posterior capsule of the hip joint may be incised, or excised, and the hip dislocated.

Indications

This approach was originally described for unipolar femoral head replacement and remains satisfactory for that indication. It is useful in posterior dislocation, particularly with fractures of the posterior column or the posterior lip.

Advantages

1. Rapid exposure through relatively bloodless planes.
2. Excellent exposure of posterior lip and posterior column of the acetabulum.

Disadvantages

1. Dependent incision, with a tendency to oedema.
2. Acetabular exposure is inferior to that of lateral approaches.
3. Increased risk of postoperative infection and/or dislocation.

Medial approach (Ludloff)

The adductor approach was described by Ludloff in 1908. He originally described a posteromedial approach and, in 1939, modified it to the present anteromedial approach.

Access

This approach gives excellent access to the lesser trochanter and the psoas tendon. It can be extended to expose the medial and inferior margins of the acetabulum and the anteroinferior capsule of the joint.

Position

The patient is placed supine, the perineum well prepared and the leg draped free.

Incision

A longitudinal incision is made over the adductor longus beginning just distal to the pubic tubercle and extending for 10 cm (Figure 1.37).

Approach

The deep fascia is incised along the posterior margin of adductor longus (Figure 1.38). Often this muscle can be released, especially if tight. The plane between adductor longus and adductor brevis is developed, adductor longus being retracted anteriorly. If the hip is now flexed, abducted and externally rotated, the lesser trochanter is brought closer to the skin and by blunt dissection in this plane it can be palpated and exposed.

The anterior branch of the obturator nerve lies on the front of adductor brevis and is protected (Figure 1.39). The iliopsoas can be divided and this exposes the anterior and inferior aspects of the capsule of the hip joint. This can be opened, if required, in a longitudinal direction. Closure is simply accomplished by resuturing the fascia and skin.

Indications

This is the approach of choice for lesions of the lesser trochanter, such as osteoid osteoma. It is a useful incision for psoas tenotomy and anterior capsulotomy where this is combined with an adductor release. It is not a recommended approach for congenital dislocation of the hip, as exposure is limited and femoral head blood supply is at risk.

Advantages

1. Minimal morbidity.
2. Direct access to lesser trochanter.

Disadvantages

1. Incision close to perineum.
2. Limited exposure of capsule of hip joint.
3. Deep incision which can make haemostasis difficult.

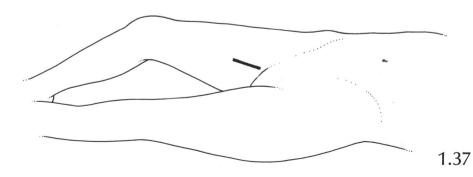

1.37

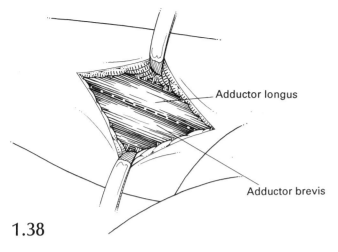

Adductor longus

Adductor brevis

1.38

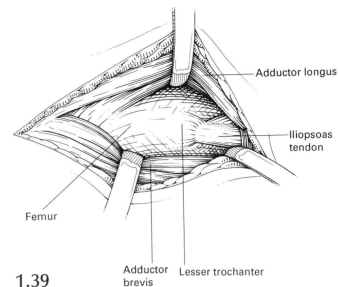

Adductor longus

Iliopsoas tendon

Femur

Adductor brevis   Lesser trochanter

1.39

References

Brackett, E. G. (1912) Study of the different approaches to the hip joint. *Boston Med. Surg.,* **CLXVI**, 235

Gibson, A. (1950) Posterior exposure of the hip joint. *J. Bone Joint Surg.,* **32B**, 183

Judet R., Judet, J. and Letournel, E. (1964) Fractures of the acetabulum: classification and surgical approaches for open reduction. *J. Bone Joint Surg.,* **46A**, 1615

Hardinge, K. (1982) The direct lateral approach to the hip. *J. Bone Joint Surg.,* **64B**, 17

Henry, A. K. (1966) *Extensile Exposure,* E. & S. Livingstone, Edinburgh

Kocher, T. (1903) *Textbook of Operative Surgery,* 2nd edn (translated from 4th German edn), Adam & Charles Black, London

Langenbeck, B. von (1874) Ueber die Schussverletzungen des Huftgelenks Arch. *Klin. Chir.,* **16**, 263

Ludloff, K. (1939) The open reduction of the congenital hip dislocation and anterior incision. *Am. J. Orthop. Surg.,* **10**, 438

McFarland, B. and Osborne, G. (1954) Approach to the hip. *J. Bone Joint Surg.,* **36B**, 364

Moore, A. T. (1957) The self-locking metal hips prosthesis. *J. Bone Joint Surg.,* **39A**, 811

Smith-Petersen, M. N. (1917) A new supra-articular approach to the hip joint. *Am. J. Orthop. Surg.,* **15**, 592

Somerville, E. W. (1953) Open reduction in congenital dislocation of the hip. *J. Bone Joint Surg.,* **35B**, 363

Watson-Jones, R. (1936) Fractures of the neck of the femur. *Br. J. Surg.,* **23**, 7878

Further reading

Charnley, J. (1979) *Low Friction Arthroplasty of the Hip,* Springer, Berlin

Rüedi, T., Hochstetter, A. H. C. and Schlumpf, R. (1984) *Surgical Approaches for Internal Fixation,* Springer, Berlin

Smith-Petersen, M. N. (1949) Approach to and exposure of the hip joint for mold arthoplasty. *J. Bone Joint Surg.,* **31A**, 40

Chapter 2

The femur

C. H. Rorabeck and J. R. Davey

RELEVANT ANATOMY

Cutaneous nerves

The lateral femoral cutaneous nerve and the genitofemoral nerves, deriving from the lumbar plexus, supply sensation to the lateral and proximal anterior aspect of the thigh respectively. Injury to either of these nerves is more likely to occur during approaches to the hip joint as opposed to exposure of the femoral shaft. The posterior cutaneous nerve arising from the sacral plexus supplies sensation to an area of skin on the posterior aspect of the thigh and leg. Injury to this nerve is most liable to occur during a posterior approach to the femur. In addition, cutaneous branches of the major peripheral nerves (femoral, obturator, tibial and common peroneal) supply sensation to the rest of the leg.

Superficial veins

LONG SAPHENOUS VEIN

The long saphenous vein, originating in the foot, enters the thigh posterior to the medial femoral condyle. It receives numerous tributaries in the thigh and becomes larger as it travels proximally. The vein becomes progressively more superficial and progressively more anterior as it ascends towards the saphenous hiatus (fossa ovalis). At this point, it penetrates the femoral sheath, emptying into the femoral vein. Injury to the long saphenous vein in the thigh is most likely to occur through the medial approach to the posterior surface of the femur in the popliteal space.

Deep nerves and vessels

SCIATIC NERVE

The sciatic nerve, a terminal branch of the sacral plexus, leaves the pelvis through the greater sciatic notch, crosses the short external rotators and leaves the gluteal region at the lower border of the quadratus femoris. In the gluteal region, the sciatic nerve is covered by the gluteus maximus. It leaves the lower border of the gluteus maximus midway between the ischial tuberosity and the greater trochanter. In the thigh, the sciatic nerve lies on the back of the adductor magnus, being applied very closely to the posterior surface of the femur. It proceeds distally under cover of the hamstrings and under the long head of biceps femoris which is the only muscle in the thigh which crosses the nerve. In the thigh, the nerve gives off muscular branches to biceps femoris, semitendinosus, semimembranosus and the ischial part of adductor magnus. All branches, with the exception of those to the short head of the biceps, come from the tibial portion of the sciatic nerve. The branches to the short head of the biceps come from the peroneal half of the nerve. While the nerve does not ordinarily divide into its two terminal branches until it reaches the popliteal region, it can sometimes appear in the back of the thigh as separate peroneal and tibial divisions.

POSTERIOR CUTANEOUS NERVE OF THE THIGH

The posterior cutaneous nerve of the thigh also arises from the sacral plexus and escapes, along with the sciatic nerve, through the greater sciatic notch. In the gluteal region, it crosses the short external rotators either on the medial side of the sciatic nerve or posterior to it, descending into the thigh deep to gluteus maximus. At this point, the posterior cutaneous nerve of the thigh is posteromedial to the sciatic nerve. In the upper part of the thigh, the nerve takes a more superficial course lying immediately underneath the deep fascia. Proximally, the posterior cutaneous nerve of the thigh lies on the long head of the biceps which separates it from the sciatic nerve. Distally, the nerve lies in the fat in the popliteal fossa. Injury to the nerve is most likely to occur during a posterior approach to the femur and care must be taken to identify the nerve once the deep fascia has been incised.

FEMORAL ARTERY

The femoral artery is the main arterial supply of the lower limb. It enters the thigh in the femoral triangle as the most lateral structure. It descends through the femoral triangle into the subsartorial canal and travels distally to end behind the femur at the junction of the middle and lower thirds, passing medial to the femur through the adductor hiatus to become the popliteal artery. Within the subsartorial canal the saphenous nerve travels with it, together with the nerve to vastus medialis. The femoral vein is initially posterior to the artery and then comes to lie posterolateral in the distal third.

The profunda femoris artery arises 3 or 4 cm below the inguinal ligament from the lateral side of the femoral artery curving posteriorly and medially. It passes behind the adductor longus and ends by piercing the adductor magnus distally as a fourth perforating artery. The femoral artery has no other significant branches in the thigh. The profunda femoris artery, on the other hand, gives off three perforating branches before ending as the fourth perforating artery. These branches pierce the posterior intermuscular septum and supply vastus intermedius as well as vastus lateralis.

Injuries to the femoral artery may occur through the medial approach to the posterior surface of the femur in the popliteal space. Occasionally, the artery can be injured at the adductor hiatus, where it is closely applied to bone, by the errant placement of a spiked lever retractor. The perforating branches of the profunda femoris artery always need to be divided during the posterolateral approach to the femur.

SURGICAL APPROACHES

- Anterolateral
- Lateral
- Posterolateral
- Posterior
- Posterior surface of femur in popliteal space
  Medial
  Lateral

Anterolateral approach (Figure 2.1(a))

Access

This approach allows access to the distal four-fifths of the anterior surface of the shaft of the femur.

Incision

With the patient supine, a vertical skin incision is made using the line joining the anterior superior iliac spine proximally and the lateral corner of the superior pole of the patella distally as a landmark (Figure 2.1(b)).

Approach

The incision is carried down through fat to expose the fascia covering the confluence of the quadriceps mechanism. Rectus femoris is identified along with vastus lateralis and the interval between these two muscles is developed (Figure 2.1(c)). The interval is best identified distally and then dissection continued proximally. The vastus lateralis is retracted laterally and the rectus femoris medially to expose the underlying vastus intermedius. The vastus intermedius can be split in line with its fibres to expose the underlying femur (Figure 2.1(e)). Care should be taken in the upper portion of the incision to identify the lateral femoral circumflex artery and nerve to vastus lateralis as illustrated in Figure 2.1(d),(e). This bundle should be retracted rather than divided. This neurovascular bundle limits the proximal extent of the approach. Distally, the incision is limited because of the confluence of the rectus femoris tendon joining vastus lateralis. The incision can, however, be extended distally by splitting this interval if need be.

Complete exposure of the middle and distal thirds of the femoral shaft can be carried out using this incision with careful retraction of the bundle containing the lateral femoral circumflex artery and nerve to vastus lateralis (Figure 2.1(e)).

Indications

This approach can be used for the treatment of fractures and tumours of the lower two-thirds of the femur.

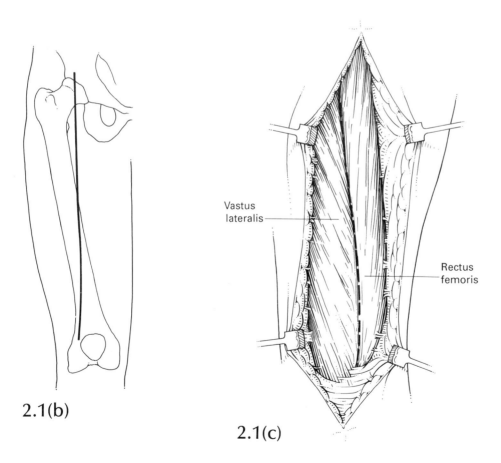

Femoral artery and vein
Sartorius
Rectus femoris
Vastus medialis
Vastus intermedius
Vastus lateralis
Femur
Adductor longus
Adductor brevis
Gracilis
Adductor magnus
Biceps femoris
Biceps femoris
Semimembranosus
Semitendinosus
Sciatic nerve

2.1(a)

2.1(b)

Vastus lateralis
Rectus femoris

2.1(c)

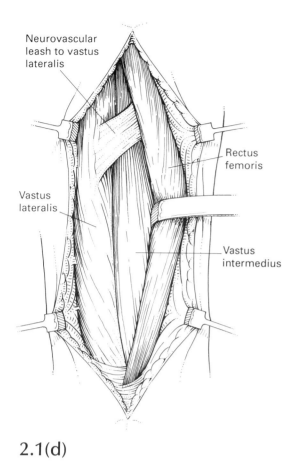

Neurovascular leash to vastus lateralis

Rectus femoris

Vastus lateralis

Vastus intermedius

2.1(d)

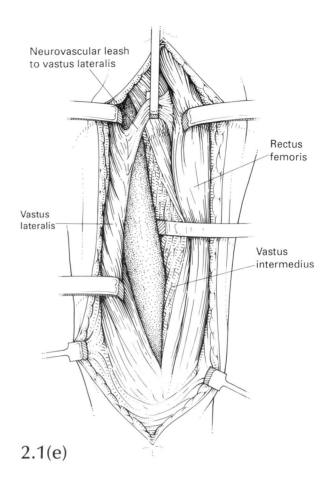

Neurovascular leash to vastus lateralis

Rectus femoris

Vastus lateralis

Vastus intermedius

2.1(e)

Lateral approach (Figure 2.2(a))

Access

The lateral approach to the femur affords access to the entire lateral and anterior surfaces of the femur from the greater trochanter proximally to the lateral femoral condyle distally. It may be extended proximally to expose the hip joint and it may be extended distally to expose the knee.

Incision

The patient is positioned supine with a sand-bag under the ipsilateral hip. The leg is prepared and draped free. A straight incision is made using the greater trochanter proximally and the lateral condyle distally as landmarks (Figure 2.2(b)). The incision may extend along all or part of this line.

Approach

The skin, subcutaneous tissue and deep fascia are incised, including the tensor fascia lata, in line with the incision (Figure 2.2(c)).

The vastus lateralis muscle is divided in line with the incision (Figure 2.2(d)). At this point, the fibres of vastus intermedius merge with those of vastus lateralis, thus the incision is carried down through fleshy vascular muscle to bone without being able to differentiate a plane between vastus lateralis and vastus intermedius. These muscles should be split in the direction of their fibres using blunt dissection to minimize bleeding.

Two important arterial branches are encountered, one proximally and one distally in this dissection. A branch of the lateral femoral circumflex artery is encountered in the proximal third and distally, at the level of the lateral femoral condyle, a branch of the superior lateral geniculate artery is identified. These should be tied and divided.

This approach is adequate to expose the entire shaft of the femur from the greater trochanter to the lateral femoral condyle.

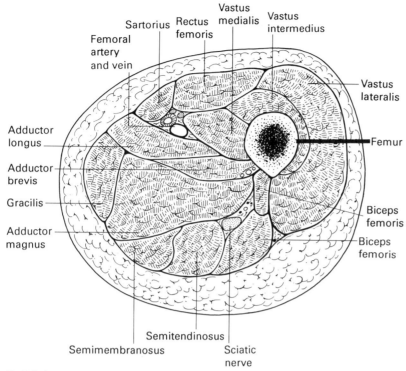

Femoral artery and vein

Sartorius

Rectus femoris

Vastus medialis

Vastus intermedius

Vastus lateralis

Femur

Adductor longus

Adductor brevis

Gracilis

Adductor magnus

Biceps femoris

Biceps femoris

Semimembranosus

Semitendinosus

Sciatic nerve

2.2(a)

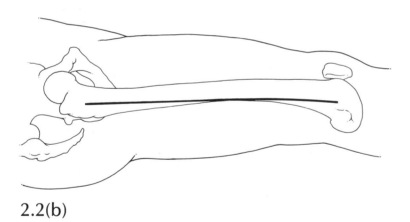

2.2(b)

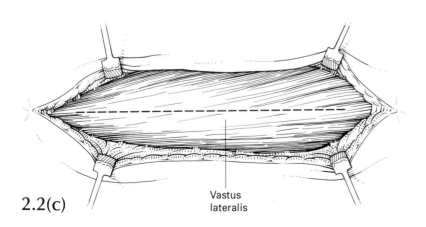

Vastus lateralis

2.2(c)

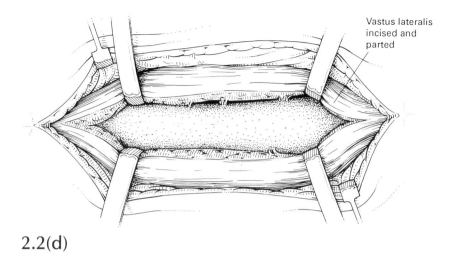

Vastus lateralis
incised and
parted

2.2(d)

Indications

Sections, or all, of this incision can be used for the treatment of fractures of any part of the femur from the hip to the knee.

Posterolateral approach (Figure 2.3(a))

Access

The posterolateral approach to the femur allows access to the lateral aspect of the femoral shaft from the origin of the vastus lateralis proximally at the level of the rough line to the lateral epicondyle distally. The incision may be extended proximally to expose the anterior aspect of the hip joint. It may also be extended distally to expose the femoral condyles and the knee joint as need be.

Incision

The patient is positioned supine with a sand-bag placed under the ipsilateral hip. The leg is prepared and draped free. The greater trochanter proximally and the lateral femoral condyle distally are used as landmarks in planning the skin incision. The incision is made in a straight line slightly posterior to these two points (Figure 2.3(b)).

Approach

Subcutaneous tissue, deep fascia and tensor fascia lata are divided in line with the incision. Care should be taken to divide the fascia lata along the anterior border of the iliotibial band.

The vastus lateralis muscle is exposed throughout the length of the incision. Two or three small retractors should then be used to retract the muscle mass as far anteriorly as possible so that the surgeon can follow the muscle posteriorly towards the point of attachment of the lateral intermuscular septum (Figure 2.3(c)).

The muscle should be detached posteriorly with blunt dissection leaving a 1.0 cm cuff of muscle tissue in front of the linea aspera. This will allow identification of the two or three perforating branches of the profunda femoris artery which are found in the distal two-thirds of this incision and which should be clamped, divided and tied (Figure 2.3(d)). If these branches are inadvertently divided, the cuff of muscle tissue will allow the operator to identify and tie them without fear of their retracting through the intermuscular septum. The bulk of the muscle is retracted anteriorly with the aid of Hohmann retractors or self-retaining retractors by either extraperiosteal or sub-periosteal dissection.

Care should be taken to avoid inadvertently perforating the lateral intermuscular septum, as damage to the sciatic nerve or the profunda femoris artery or vein may occur because of their close proximity to the intermuscular septum.

Indications

This incision can be used in the treatment of fractures and tumours of the femur. Its distal extension is used in the treatment of supracondylar fractures (see Chapter 3).

This approach is less damaging to the quadriceps femoris than the lateral and anterolateral approaches to the femur, and there is less likelihood of restriction of knee flexion from muscle scarring.

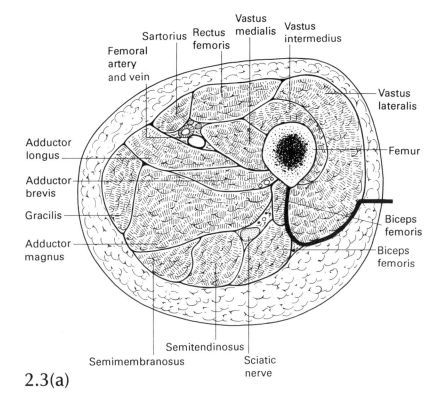

2.3(a)

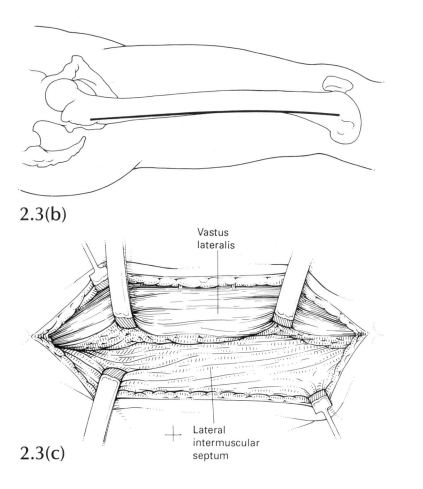

2.3(b)

2.3(c)

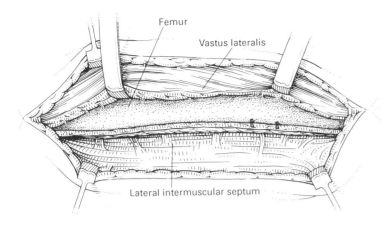

Femur

Vastus lateralis

Lateral intermuscular septum

2.3(d)

Posterior approach (Figure 2.4(a))

Access

The posterior approach to the femur allows access to the entire posterior surface of the diaphysis, although it is best suited for the middle and proximal thirds. In exposure of the distal third of the posterior surface of the femur, dissection must be carried out along the medial side of the long head of biceps and this can be technically treacherous.

Incision

The patient is positioned prone between bolsters so as to avoid pressure on the abdomen. The leg is prepared and draped free. A straight incision is used along the line extending from the mid-point of the gluteal fold to the mid-point of the popliteal fossa distally (Figure 2.4(b)). Care must be taken to avoid injury to the posterior cutaneous nerve of the thigh where it lies immediately underneath the deep fascia.

Approach

The skin and subcutaneous tissue are divided and after incising the deep fascia, the posterior cutaneous nerve of the thigh is identified. The long head of biceps is identified crossing the incision laterally and the semitendinosus and semimembranosus medially (Figure 2.4(c)). The lateral edge of the long head of the biceps is the key to the exposure.

The long head of biceps is retracted medially and the interval between the short head and the long head is developed, care being taken to avoid the branch of the sciatic nerve to the short head of the biceps (Figure 2.4(d)). The sciatic nerve must always be identified in this approach lying deep to the long head of the biceps, coursing distally and medially.

Dissection along the lateral side of the long head of biceps, between it and the short head and vastus lateralis, will provide exposure to the proximal two-thirds of the posterior surface of the femoral shaft. The long head of biceps muscle crosses the back of the femur in the distal third of the thigh and therefore to expose the distal third of the diaphysis of the posterior surface of the femur, dissection must be carried along the medial side of the long head of biceps muscle going between it and the semitendinosus (Figure 2.4(e)).

This is a potentially dangerous dissection insofar as the sciatic nerve courses the length of the incision and must be identified, and in the extreme distal end of the incision the popliteal vein and artery come into view from the medial side. Injury to any of these three structures can be avoided only through careful and meticulous dissection.

The nerve supply to the long head of biceps and semitendinosus come off the sciatic nerve at the junction of the middle and distal thirds and therefore can also be injured in this incision (Figure 2.4(e)).

Indications

Exposure of femoral shaft fractures, particularly when posterior structures have been injured by the fracture. Tumours of the posterior aspect of the femur and lesions of the sciatic nerve can be best explored by this route.

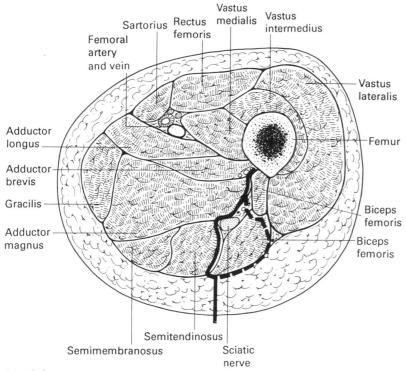

2.4(a)

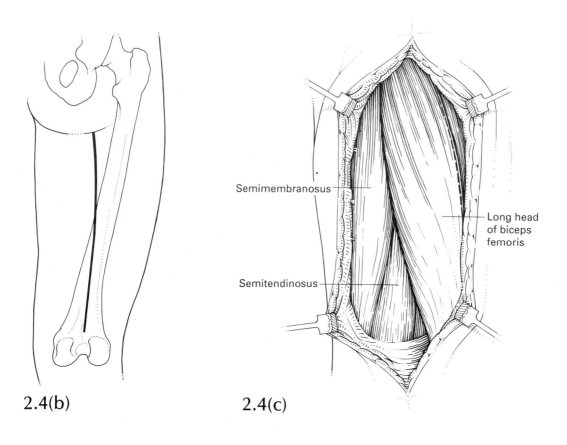

2.4(b)   2.4(c)

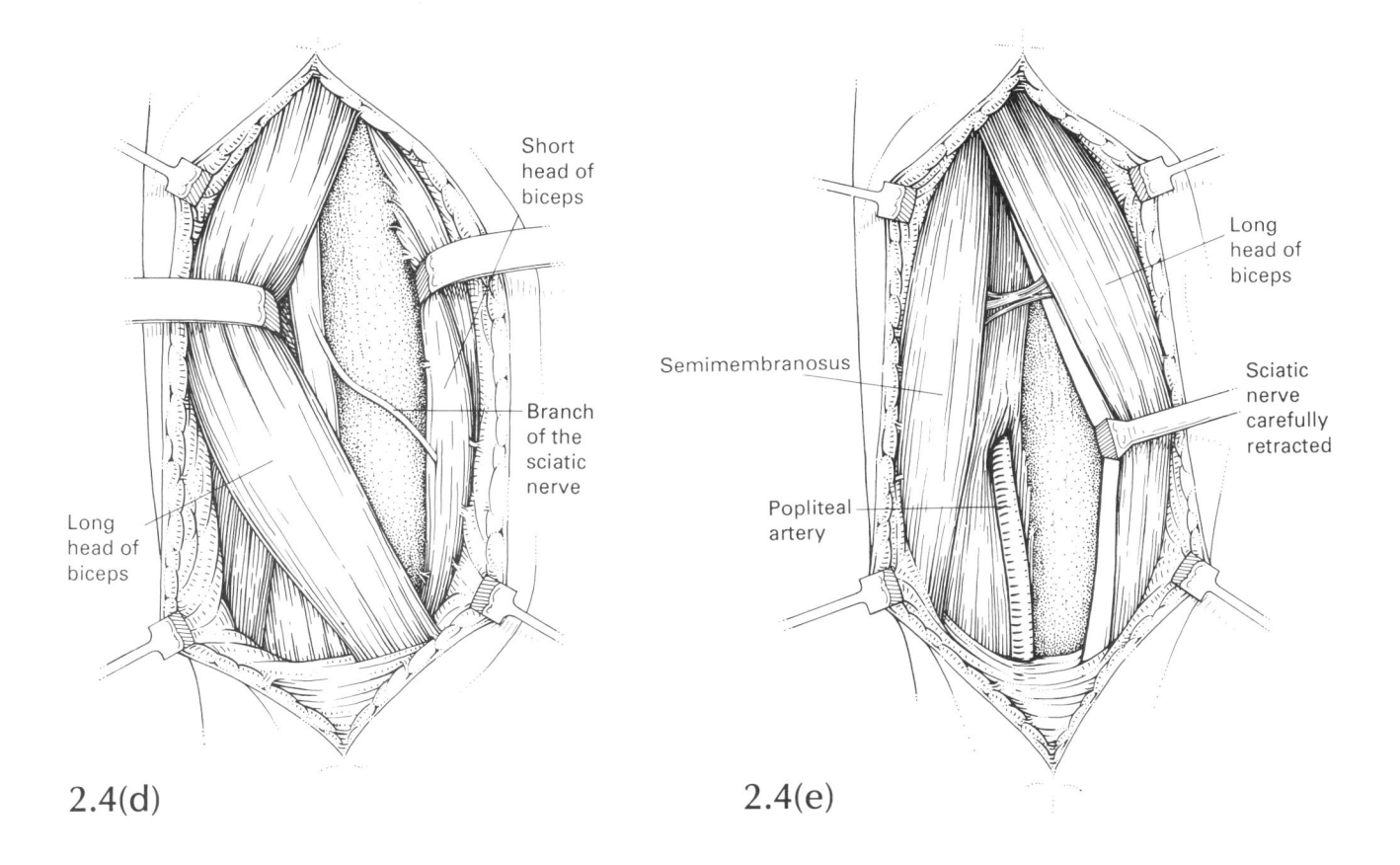

Short
head of
biceps

Branch
of the
sciatic
nerve

Long
head of
biceps

Long
head of
biceps

Sciatic
nerve
carefully
retracted

Semimembranosus

Popliteal
artery

2.4(d)

2.4(e)

Medial approach to the posterior surface of the femur in the popliteal space

Access

The medial approach to the posterior surface of the femur allows limited access to this region.

Incision

The patient is positioned supine with the leg prepared and draped free. The incision is planned to follow the tendon of the adductor magnus. Thus, the adductor tubercle is identified and marked and the course of the adductor tendon is followed proximally. The skin incision forms a straight line along the posterior border of the tendon of adductor magnus extending from the tubercle as far proximal as need be (Figure 2.5(a)).

Approach

After dividing the skin and subcutaneous tissue, the anterior edge of the sartorius muscle is identified. This anatomical landmark is best found distally in the incision (Figure 2.5(b)).

With the knee flexed the fascia is incised along the anterior border of the sartorius which then falls posteriorly, exposing the tendon of the adductor magnus muscle inserting into the adductor tubercle anteriorly (Figure 2.5(c)).

The adductor magnus muscle and tendon are retracted posteriorly and vastus lateralis is retracted anteriorly to expose the femur (Figure 2.5(d)).

The neurovascular bundle will be lying in the popliteal space directly behind the femur at this level and if necessary can be exposed through this incision by dissecting behind adductor magnus and its tendon.

Indications

It may be utilized to expose an osteochondroma or other neoplastic lesion of bone in this area. The approach is also useful to expose the neurovascular bundle in the event of an arterial injury complicating a distal femoral fracture, and extended distally for posterior cruciate exposure (see Chapter 3).

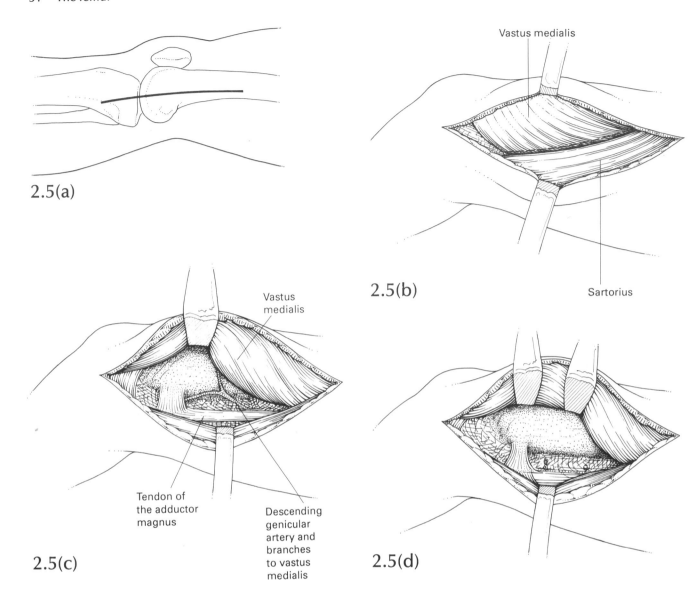

2.5(a)

2.5(b)

Vastus medialis

Sartorius

2.5(c)

Vastus medialis

Tendon of the adductor magnus

Descending genicular artery and branches to vastus medialis

2.5(d)

Lateral approach to the posterior surface of the femur in the popliteal space

Access

This approach allows access to the back of the knee and the posterior surface of the distal one-fifth of the femoral shaft.

Incision

The patient is positioned supine with a sand-bag under the ipsilateral hip and with the table slightly tilted towards the opposite side. Alternatively, the patient may be positioned in a straight lateral position with the leg prepared and draped free. With the knee in an extended position, a straight skin incision should be made along an imaginary line drawn between the head of the fibula and the greater trochanter. It should parallel the posterior border of the iliotibial band (Figure 2.6(a)).

Approach

After the skin incision has been made, the posterior border of the iliotibial band is identified and incised so that the iliotibial band can be retracted anteriorly (Figure 2.6(b)).

The iliotibial band has to be separated from the short head of the biceps muscle. After developing that interval

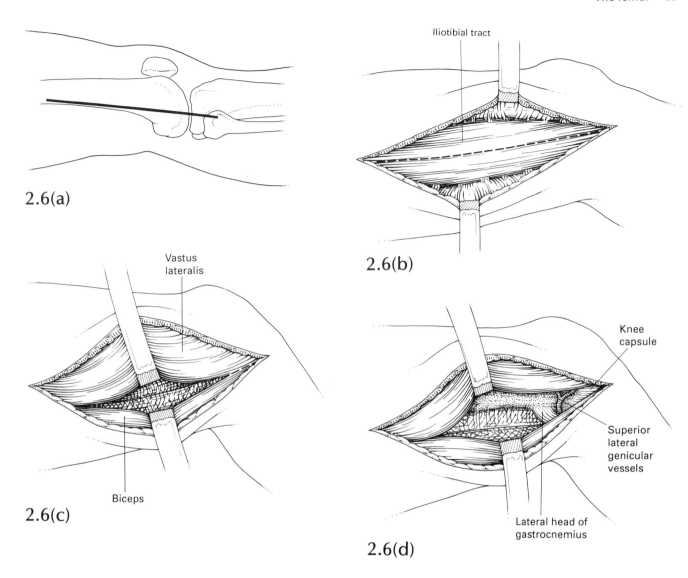

2.6(a)

2.6(b)

Iliotibial tract

2.6(c)

Vastus
lateralis

Biceps

2.6(d)

Knee
capsule

Superior
lateral
genicular
vessels

Lateral head of
gastrocnemius

the short head of biceps is retracted posteriorly and the iliotibial band anteriorly.

Dissection is continued behind the lateral intermuscular septum to bone.

The short head and long head of the biceps muscle are retracted posteriorly to expose the shaft of the femur and the posterior border of the femur in the popliteal fossa (Figure 2.6(c), (d)). This is helped by flexing the knee. The surgeon will encounter branches of the lateral superior geniculate vessels which must be divided and tied.

Care must be taken with retraction of the neurovascular structures in the popliteal fossa. The common peroneal nerve can be injured where it lies immediately along the medial edge of the long head of biceps.

A blunt retractor should always be used to expose the popliteal surface of the femur through this lateral approach.

Indications

It is used most commonly in knee ligament reconstructions, particularly with 'over the top' repairs for anterolateral or posterolateral rotatory instability. It also approaches to the distal one-fifth of the femur, particularly when simultaneous access to the intercondylar area is required, as, for example, in anterior cruciate ligament reconstructions.

Further reading

Bosworth, D. M. (1944) Posterior approach to the femur. *J. Bone Joint Surg.*, **26**, 687

Crenshaw, A. H. (1980) Surgical approaches. In *Campbell's Operative Orthopaedics* (eds A. S. Edmonson and A. H. Crenshaw), C. V. Mosby, St Louis

Darrach, W. (1945) Surgical approaches for surgery of the extremities. *Am. J. Surg.*, **67**, 237

Grant, J. C. B. (1972) *Grant's Atlas of Anatomy,* Williams and Wilkins, Baltimore

Harty, M. and Joyce, J. J. (1963) Surgical approaches to the hip and femur. *J. Bone Joint Surg.*, **45A**, 175

Henry, A. K. (1924–25) Exposure of the humerus and femoral shaft. *Br. J. Surg.*, **12**, 84

Hollinshead, W. H. (1982) *Anatomy for Surgeons,* vol. 3, Harper and Row, Philadelphia

Marcy, G. H. (1947) Posterolateral approach to the femur. *J. Bone Joint Surg.*, **29**, 676

Müller, M. E., Allgöwer, M., Schneider, R. *et al.* (1979) *Manual of Internal Fixation,* Springer, Berlin

Romanes, C. J. (1976) *Cunningham's Manual of Practical Anatomy,* vol. 1, Oxford University Press, Oxford

Thompson, J. E. (1918) Anatomical methods of approach in operations on the long bones of the extremities. *Ann. Surg.*, **68**, 309

Chapter 3

The knee

A. J. Hall

RELEVANT ANATOMY

Planning incisions around the knee should be based on sound anatomical knowledge. Anteriorly, the blood supply and venous drainage are important considerations for subsequent healing. Superficial nerves, particularly the infrapatellar branch of the saphenous nerve, should be preserved whenever possible to avoid painful neuromas.

When planning a limited approach to the knee joint it is always wise to consider how the wound could be extended should a wider exposure become necessary.

Posteriorly, the attachments of muscles and the presence of major neurovascular structures dictate the approach, although they need not restrict access providing sufficient care is taken to plan the exposure required.

Arteries

The popliteal artery is the continuation of the femoral artery after it has passed through the opening in the adductor magnus at the junction of the middle and lower thirds of the thigh. Just before entering the opening in adductor magnus, the femoral artery gives off the descending genicular artery (Figure 3.1(b)), which in turn gives off the saphenous branch to the medial side of the front of the knee, before it passes, within the substance of the vastus medialis, to the medial side of the knee to anastomose with the medial superior genicular artery. It also gives off articular branches, one of which crosses

laterally, above the patella, to form an anastomotic arch with the lateral superior genicular artery.

The popliteal artery reaches the mid-line posteriorly and runs down to the lower border of popliteus, where it divides into anterior and posterior tibial arteries (Figure 3.1(a)).

In the popliteal fossa the artery gives rise to several large branches.

Medially there are two or three superior muscular branches to the adductor magnus and hamstrings, anastomosing with the terminal branches of the profunda femoris artery. The medial superior genicular artery (Figure 3.1(a)–(c)) runs between the semimembranosus and semitendinosus muscles and the medial head of gastrocnemius, beneath the tendon of adductor magnus, to enter the vastus medialis, which it supplies, and gives off a branch to anastomose with the terminal branches of the descending genicular and the medial inferior genicular arteries.

One of the two sural arteries (Figure 3.1(a)) is also found on the medial side where it supplies gastrocnemius and soleus.

The medial inferior genicular artery (Figure 3.1(a)) arises from the popliteal artery and passes around the medial condyle of the tibia, deep to the medial head of gastrocnemius, along the upper border of popliteus (which it supplies). It then passes deep to the medial collateral ligament, at the front of which it divides into branches which anastomose with the lateral inferior and medial superior genicular arteries (Figure 3.1(b),(c)).

Laterally, there are also three branches of the popliteal artery. The lateral superior genicular artery (Figure 3.1(a)) passes beneath the biceps femoris tendon and divides into a superficial branch, which supplies vastus lateralis and anastomoses with the descending branch of the lateral circumflex femoral artery, and a deep branch which

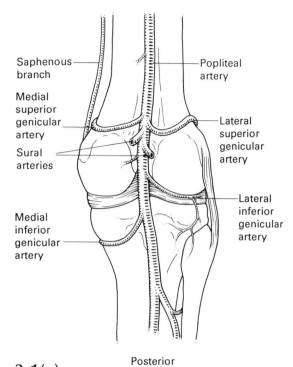

3.1(a)   Posterior

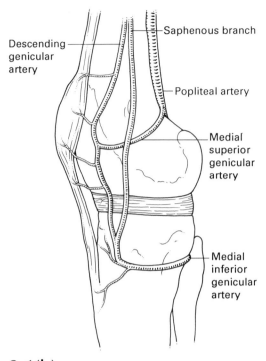

3.1(b)   Medial

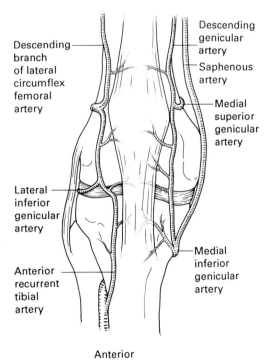

3.1(c)   Anterior

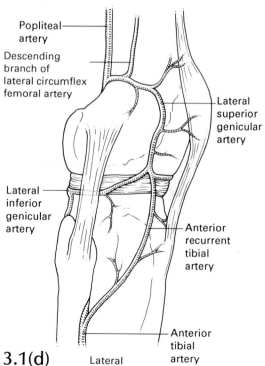

3.1(d)   Lateral

anastomoses with the medial superior genicular artery and forms an arch across the front of the femur with the descending genicular artery (Figure 3.1(d)).

The other sural artery supplies (Figure 3.1(a)) the lateral head of gastrocnemius.

The lateral inferior genicular artery runs laterally across popliteus, then forwards, deep to the lateral ligament, to divide into branches which anastomose with the medial inferior genicular artery, lateral superior genicular and anterior tibial recurrent arteries (Figure 3.1(a),(c),(d)).

The middle genicular artery is a small branch arising from the front of the popliteal artery at the level of the knee joint. It pierces the oblique posterior ligament and supplies the cruciate ligaments and synovial membrane of the knee joint.

At the distal border of popliteus the popliteal artery divides into the anterior and posterior tibial arteries.

Caution. Occasionally this division takes place at the upper border of popliteus, in which case the anterior tibial artery descends in front of the popliteus.

Veins

The deep veins accompany the arteries and their branches. The popliteal vein is formed by the junction of the anterior and posterior tibial veins at the lower border of popliteus. At first it is medial to the popliteal artery, then between the heads of gastrocnemius it comes to lie superficial to it and above the knee it becomes postero-lateral to it (Figure 3.2(a)). Its tributaries are the short saphenous vein and the veins corresponding to the branches of the popliteal artery.

The long saphenous vein, the longest vein in the body, crosses the knee joint on the posteromedial aspect. It is accompanied at the knee by the saphenous branch of the descending genicular artery.

The vein has many tributaries and communicates freely with the short saphenous system.

Note. The short saphenous vein occasionally ends below the knee in the long saphenous vein or in the deep muscular veins of the calf.

Nerves

The saphenous nerve is the largest cutaneous branch of the femoral nerve. As it traverses Hunter's canal, it crosses from the lateral to the medial side of the femoral artery. At the lower end of the canal, it leaves through the aponeurotic roof to accompany the saphenous branch of the descending genicular artery. It descends on the

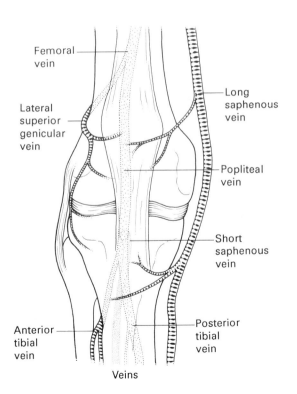

Veins

3.2(a)

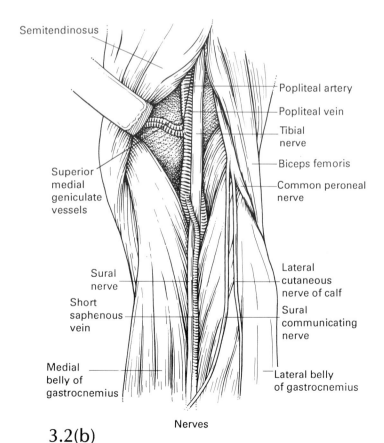

Nerves

3.2(b)

medial side of the knee between sartorius and gracilis, pierces the deep fascia just below the knee to become subcutaneous, and then descends along the medial border of the tibia to the lower third of the leg where it divides into two branches. Its infrapatellar branch is given off after leaving the adductor canal. It pierces sartorius and the deep fascia and supplies the skin in front of the patella.

The sciatic nerve divides into tibial and common peroneal nerves in the lower third of the thigh.

The tibial nerve (Figure 3.2(b)) (derived from the ventral branches of the anterior primary rami of L4, L5 and S1–3) descends through the middle of the popliteal fossa to the lower border of the popliteus muscle, where it passes deep to the arch of soleus with the popliteal artery.

In the popliteal fossa it lies lateral to the vessels. At the level of the knee joint it lies superficial to the vessels and below the joint crosses to their medial side.

There are usually three articular branches accompanying the medial superior, medial inferior and middle genicular arteries.

Muscular branches arise from the nerve to supply gastrocnemius, plantaris, soleus and popliteus.

The sural nerve descends between the two heads of gastrocnemius, pierces the deep fascia below the knee and is joined by the sural communicating branch of the common peroneal nerve (Figure 3.2(b)).

The common peroneal nerve (Figure 3.2(b)), about half the size of the tibial and derived from dorsal branches of anterior primary rami of L4, L5 and S1, S2, descends obliquely along the lateral side of the popliteal fossa to the head of the fibula, close to the medial margin of the biceps femoris muscle and tendon. It lies between the biceps femoris tendon and lateral head of gastrocnemius, then winds around the lateral surface of the neck of the fibula, deep to peroneus longus. It gives off three articular branches; one accompanies the lateral superior genicular artery and one the lateral inferior genicular artery. The third branch is given off near the point of division of the common peroneal nerve and ascends, with the anterior recurrent tibial artery, to supply the anterolateral capsule of the knee joint.

There are two cutaneous branches of the common peroneal nerve. The lateral cutaneous nerve of the calf is given off in the high popliteal fossa, where it pierces the roof of the fossa over the lateral head of gastrocnemius and supplies the skin on the anterior, posterior and lateral surfaces of the proximal part of the leg. The sural communicating branch (Figure 3.2(b)) arises near the head of the fibula and runs obliquely across the lateral head of gastrocnemius to the middle of the leg, where it joins the sural nerve. It may descend as a separate branch as far as the heel.

Note. The posterior branch of the obturator nerve gives off an articular branch to the knee which descends on the popliteal artery and pierces the oblique posterior ligament of the knee to reach the capsule.

SURGICAL APPROACHES: ARTHROSCOPIC INCISIONS

At first sight the inclusion of arthroscopic incisions in this chapter might seem irrelevant but, as is the case with many surgical procedures, the ease with which an operation is carried out frequently depends upon the surgical approach and this certainly applies to arthroscopic surgery.

- Anterolateral
- Anteromedial
- Central (Gillquist and Hagberg)
- Suprapatellar
- Posteromedial
- Posterolateral

Vertical or horizontal incisions?

The lines of cleavage (Langer's lines) around the knee might suggest a horizontal incision but the planes of the tight medial and lateral compartments of the knee are horizontal and therefore a poorly placed horizontal incision gives no room for manoeuvre, whereas a vertical incision can easily be extended to provide the access required (Figure 3.3).

ANTEROLATERAL ARTHROSCOPIC APPROACH (Figure 3.3)

The knee should be distended with saline before making the stab incision, in order to achieve a 'cleaner' penetration through the synovium of the knee. The thumb is then placed in the angle between the patellar tendon and the joint line of the flexed knee and the incision is made *above* the thumb (Figure 3.3). The common mistake is to make the incision too low so that the arthroscope is inserted uncomfortably close to the anterior attachment of the lateral meniscus.

Indications

Standard incision for routine arthroscopy of the knee.

ANTEROMEDIAL ARTHROSCOPIC INCISION (Figure 3.4)

This incision is best made whilst observing the entry of the knife arthroscopically. The point of entry should be slightly higher than that of the lateral incision to facilitate access to the region of the posterior horn of the meniscus.

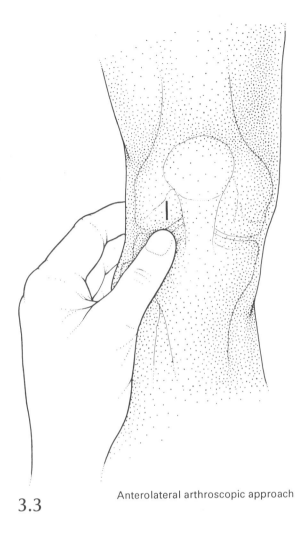

3.3   Anterolateral arthroscopic approach

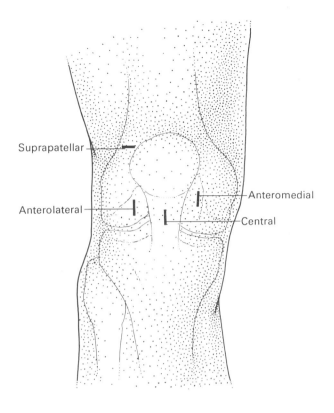

Arthroscopic incision

3.4

Indications

Insertion of probes and hooks for diagnostic arthroscopy and instruments for surgery. An alternative insertion of the arthroscope for viewing the lateral meniscus.

CENTRAL ARTHROSCOPIC APPROACH (Gillquist and Hagberg) (Figure 3.4)

A central approach can be used for routine examination of the knee as an alternative to the anterolateral insertion.

The knee should be flexed to 60 degrees and the stab incision made in the mid-line 1 cm below the lower pole of the patella, down to (but not into) the tendon. A sharp trocar is then used to penetrate the tendon in a slightly upward direction. As the joint is entered the knee is extended, the blunt obturator replaces the sharp obturator, and the tip of the instrument is redirected towards the suprapatellar pouch prior to inserting the telescope.

Indications

Routine arthroscopic examination of the knee with better access to the posterior compartment than the anterolateral approach. Not recommended for insertion of instruments.

SUPRAPATELLAR ARTHROSCOPIC INCISIONS (Figure 3.4)

The suprapatellar pouch is so large that the possibilities for arthroscopic stab incisions are almost limitless. The most useful position is immediately lateral to the upper pole of the patella.

Indications

Insertion of operating instruments for anterior compartment lesions, particularly those affecting the patella, infrapatellar fat pad and the medial synovial shelf. Alternatively, the arthroscope can be inserted through this approach whilst operating through the anterolateral approach on anterior joint structures. The patellofemoral joint, medial synovial shelf, the fat pad and anterior horns of medial and lateral menisci can all be seen.

POSTEROMEDIAL ARTHROSCOPIC APPROACH

This approach is sometimes required to complete the examination of the medial compartment. The stab incision is made with the knee flexed to 90 degrees at a point behind the medial femoral condyle and above the tibial plateau. This approach is more difficult than it sounds and it is best to insert a needle at the proposed site for the incision. If there is free flow of saline from the joint, the incision can be made along the needle.

Indications

Arthroscopic inspection of the posteromedial compartment, including the posterior cruciate ligament and the posterior aspect of the medial meniscus. Instruments may be inserted through the incision whilst the cavity is viewed through a 70 degree telescope inserted through the intercondylar notch from the front of the knee.

POSTEROLATERAL ARTHROSCOPIC APPROACH

Rarely needed, this approach tends to be more traumatic than the posteromedial approach. It is best made 'under direct vision' using the 70 degree telescope inserted from the front of the joint; a needle is inserted posterolaterally and when in the optimum position, as viewed through the telescope, the stab incision is made alongside the needle.

Indications

This approach is used mainly for the removal of loose bodies from the posterolateral compartment and for arthroscopic synovectomy.

Positioning for arthroscopic approaches

The patient is supine on the operating table. A pneumatic tourniquet is applied as high as possible on the thigh to avoid tethering the muscles of the thigh. Some surgeons use a padded thigh clamp in order to improve the leverage on the joint during arthroscopic surgery, but caution should be exercised if these devices are used as there have been reports of ligament damage.

After suitable skin preparation the drapes are applied so as to leave the leg free. Preliminary distension of the joint is carried out with the knee extended. The trocar and cannula are inserted with the knee slightly flexed. The anterior compartment is examined with the knee extended. The medial compartment is examined with the

knee flexed. The operator can sit with the foot between his knees and impart a valgus and external rotation strain to the knee joint in order to improve access. If the posteromedial part of the medial meniscus cannot be easily seen the knee should be extended whilst a valgus strain is applied.

The lateral compartment can be examined in the same way but with a varus strain applied to the knee. Alternatively the knee can be flexed to 90 degrees and the heel placed on the operating table so that the knee falls outwards, allowing the surgeon to stand whilst gravity produces the required varus strain for access. Under these circumstances the arthroscope should be inserted through the anteromedial incision.

SURGICAL APPROACHES: OPEN APPROACHES

- Anteromedial
- Anterior (Insall)
- Posterior (Brackett and Osgood, Putti and Abbott)
- Medial and posteromedial
- Lateral
    Bruser
    To distal femur (Rüedi, von Hochstetter and Schlumpf)
    Parapatellar to knee and proximal tibia (Rüedi, von Hochstetter and Schlumpf)
- Posteromedial (Henderson)
- Posterolateral (Henderson)
- Skin incisions above the knee
    Median parapatellar (von Langenbeck and Payr)
    Oblique parapatellar (Erkes)
- Incisions interfering with extensor mechanism
- Incisions dividing the patella
- Incisions for meniscectomy
- Utility incisions

Anteromedial approach

Access

The anteromedial approach gives access to the whole of the front of the knee, including the suprapatellar pouch, the medial and lateral compartments and intercondylar region. In joint replacement further access is provided by division of the cruciate ligaments, which makes it possible to dislocate the knee.

Positioning

The patient is supine on the operating table. A pneumatic tourniquet is applied as high as possible so as to minimize compression of the thigh muscles which would otherwise

restrict mobility of the knee. After suitable skin preparation, the leg is draped free. The incision is made with the leg extended but once the capsule has been opened the knee is fully flexed whilst the patella is everted. During the operation the knee may have to be flexed and extended several times. It is important to remember however that when the knee is extended the neurovascular bundle is very close to the joint posteriorly and powered or sharp instruments should only be directed towards the back of the knee when it is flexed.

Incision (Figure 3.5)

A slightly curved skin incision starts from the mid-line, a hand's breadth above the patella, skirting the medial edge of the patella to the medial side of the tibial tubercle. A straight mid-line incision is preferred by some surgeons.

Approach

The fat and subcutaneous fascia are incised in the line of the skin incision. At the level of the deep fascia the quadriceps tendon is exposed superiorly by lateral dissection. The medial border of the patella is exposed by slight medial dissection and at the lower end the incision is over the medial border of the patellar tendon. The capsule of the knee joint can then be incised without damaging any muscle (Figure 3.6(a)–(c)).

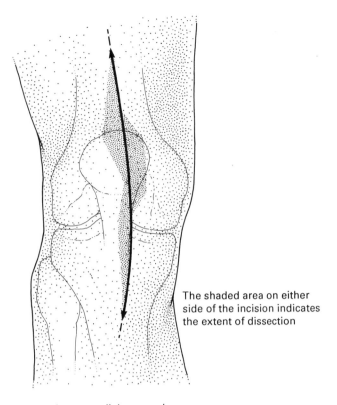

The shaded area on either side of the incision indicates the extent of dissection

Anteromedial approach

3.5

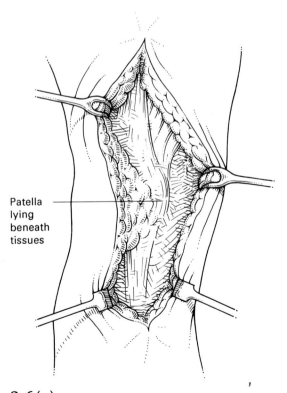

Patella lying beneath tissues

3.6(a)

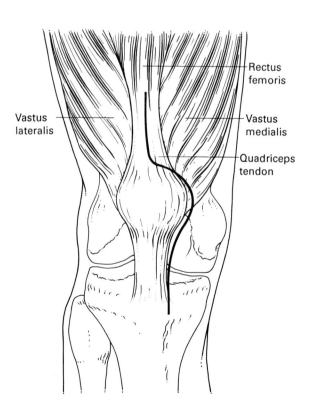

Rectus femoris

Vastus lateralis

Vastus medialis

Quadriceps tendon

3.6(b)

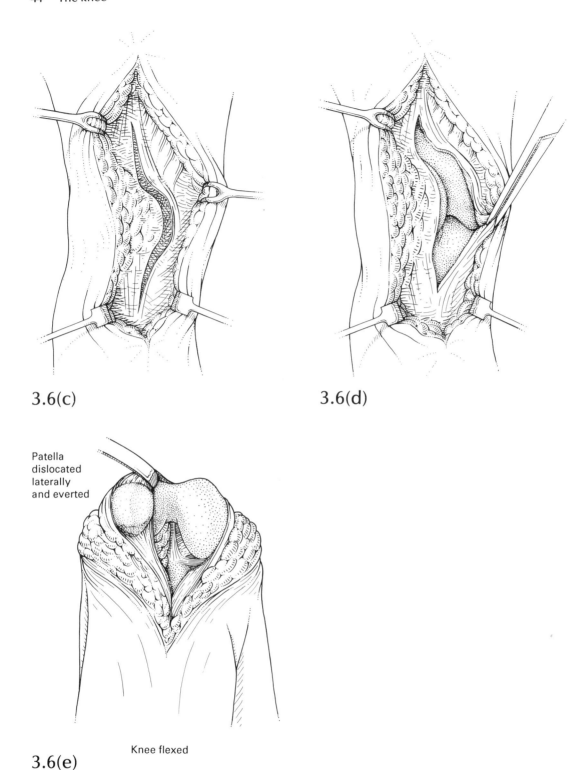

3.6(c)

3.6(d)

Patella
dislocated
laterally
and everted

Knee flexed

3.6(e)

The incision in the quadriceps tendon should be in line with its fibres. At the superomedial pole of the patella the tendon is detached, leaving a very small margin for closure. The deep incision then passes along the medial border of the patella until the patellar tendon is reached, when it descends along its medial edge to the level of the tibial tubercle (Figure 3.6(c),(d)).

At this stage the knee is flexed whilst the patella is everted and dislocated laterally (Figure 3.6(d),(e)).

Access is improved on the lateral side by cleanly removing the infrapatellar fat pad from the patellar tendon (Figure 3.7) and on the medial side by sharp dissection of the combined periosteum and fascia over the medial flare of the tibia (Figure 3.8(a)). In joint replacement surgery,

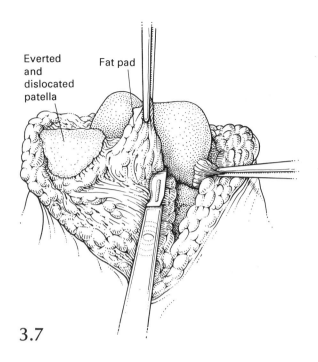

Everted and dislocated patella   Fat pad

3.7

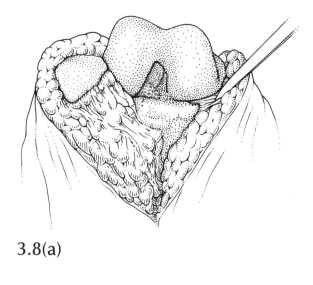

3.8(a)

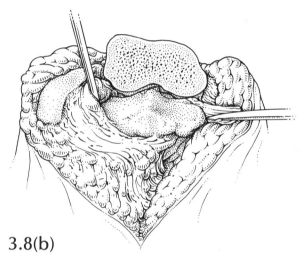

3.8(b)

further access to the joint can be obtained by division of the cruciate ligaments which permits a degree of subluxation, depending on the state of the collateral ligament.

In joint replacement, removal of the joint surfaces allows access to the posterior compartment of the knee joint (Figure 3.8(b)).

Indications

The anteromedial approach to the knee is the incision of choice for anterior synovectomy and knee joint replacement.

Anterior approach (Insall)

Access

This approach affords excellent exposure to the anterior knee joint. The incision heals well, often with a better scar than the anteromedial approach and there is a slightly smaller area of sensory denervation over the front of the knee.

Positioning

The patient is supine on the operating table. A pneumatic tourniquet is applied as high as possible so as to minimize compression of the thigh muscles which would otherwise restrict mobility of the knee. After suitable skin preparation, the leg is draped free. The incision is made with the leg extended but once the capsule has been opened the knee is fully flexed whilst the patella is everted. During the operation the knee may have to be flexed and extended several times. It is important to remember however that when the knee is extended the neurovascular bundle is very close to the joint posteriorly and powered or sharp instruments should only be directed towards the back of the knee when it is flexed.

Incision

A curved lateral parapatellar incision is made through skin and subcutaneous tissue to the deep fascia (Figure 3.9(a),(b)).

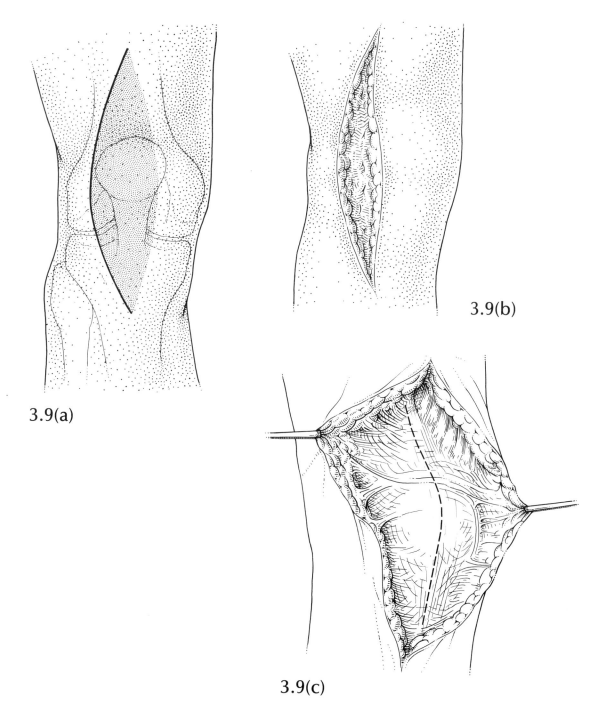

3.9(a)

3.9(b)

3.9(c)

The skin and subcutaneous tissue are now dissected medially to expose the extensor mechanism. Starting 8 cm above the patella, the quadriceps tendon is split in the mid-line and the incision is continued distally over the patella and into the patellar tendon as far as the tibial tubercle (Figure 3.9(c)). The longitudinal fibres of the quadriceps tendon are now carefully separated from the medial half of the patella preserving a substantial layer of tissue (Figure 3.10(a)). The synovium is then divided along the medial border of the patella and into the suprapatellar pouch. The infrapatellar fat pad is divided in the mid-line.

The patella is now dislocated laterally and the medial half of the quadriceps tendon is retracted medially as the knee is flexed (Figure 3.10(b)).

Indications

Joint debridement, anterior synovectomy and total knee replacement. This approach is superior to the split patellar approach of Jones and Brackett which is not recommended, due to the difficulty of accurate restoration of patellar congruity.

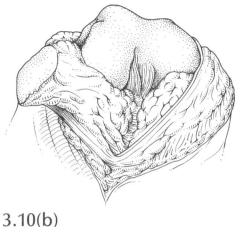

3.10(b)

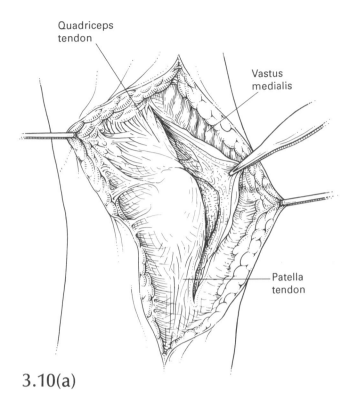

Quadriceps
tendon

Vastus
medialis

Patella
tendon

3.10(a)

Posterior approach (Brackett and Osgood, Putti, Abbott)

Access

This approach provides access to the posterior capsule of the knee joint, the posterior aspects of the femoral and tibial condyles, the posterior compartments of the knee (including the posterior parts of the menisci) and the origin of the posterior cruciate ligament. Care should be taken to protect and preserve the vital structures during this approach.

Positioning

The patient should be prone with adequate cushioning to allow free movement of the abdomen and slight flexion of the knee.

A high pneumatic tourniquet should be applied. It is often easier to do this before the patient is turned over onto the face.

The leg is draped free after adequate skin preparation.

Incision (Figure 3.11)

A gently curving incision starts posteromedially over the semitendinosus muscle, about 8cm above the joint crease, following the tendon of semitendinosus to the

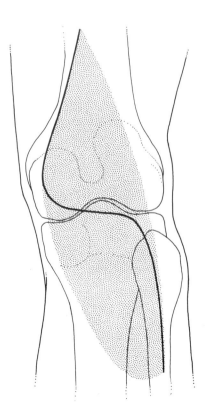

Posterior approach.
The shaded area represents
the extent of dissection of flaps

3.11

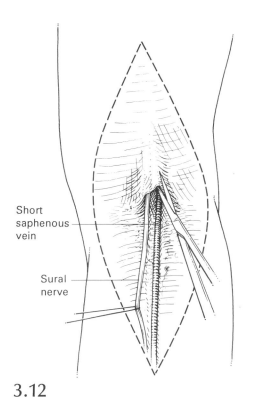

3.12

level of the joint, then passes laterally across the posterior aspect of the joint for about 5 cm before descending over the lateral belly of gastrocnemius for a further 8 cm.

Approach

Skin and subcutaneous tissue are reflected to expose the popliteal fascia. The sural nerve is identified beneath the fascia and between the two heads of gastrocnemius; it is the main guide for the dissection. On the lateral side of the nerve, the short saphenous vein perforates the popliteal fascia to join the popliteal vein in the middle of the fossa.

The sural nerve is traced to its origin from the tibial nerve (Figure 3.12). Once this nerve has been identified the dissection can be completed safely. The tibial nerve is traced distally, exposing the branches to the two heads of gastrocnemius, the plantaris and the soleus muscles. These branches are accompanied by arteries and veins.

The tibial nerve is cleared proximally to the apex of the fossa where it is joined by the common peroneal nerve to form the sciatic nerve. Next, expose the common peroneal nerve distally along the medial border of the biceps muscle and tendon and protect the lateral cutaneous nerve of the calf and the sural communicating branch (Figure 3.13). The popliteal artery and vein are now exposed lying directly anterior and medial to the tibial nerve. Gently retract the artery and vein to locate the superior medial and superior lateral genicular vessels,

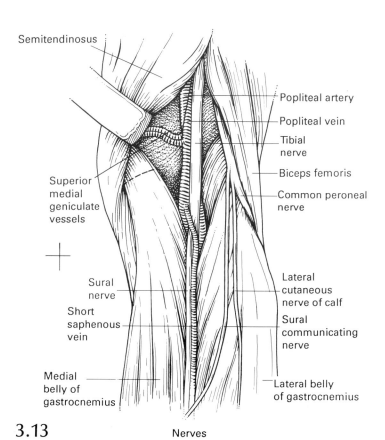

3.13   Nerves

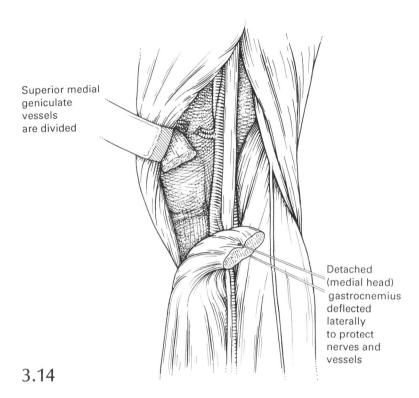

Superior medial geniculate vessels are divided

Detached (medial head) gastrocnemius deflected laterally to protect nerves and vessels

3.14

passing beneath the hamstrings just proximal to the heads of origin of the gastrocnemius muscle.

Whilst retracting the semimembranosus muscle medially, the medial head of gastrocnemius is detached close to its origin (Figure 3.14) and turned laterally to protect and retract the popliteal vessels and nerves. If greater access is needed the superior medial genicular vessels may be ligated and divided. Usually if access to the posterior cruciate ligament is required, the middle genicular vessels should be ligated and divided and as these are so short, great care is needed at this stage.

Exposure of the posterolateral aspect of the joint is achieved by detaching the lateral head of gastrocnemius, but care should be taken to avoid damage to the common peroneal nerve by retractors.

Once the large vessels and nerves are retracted the floor of the popliteal fossa is exposed and access can be gained to the structures in the posterior knee joint.

Indications

Repairs of the posterior cruciate ligament and posterior knee capsule. Removal of tumours in the popliteal fossa. Access to the posterior aspect of the proximal tibia, particularly for fractures of the posterior tibial spine associated with cruciate ligament avulsion.

Medial and posteromedial approach

Access

This approach gives access to the medial ligament, the posteromedial capsule, the posterior oblique ligament and can also be extended to expose the posterior cruciate ligament.

Incision

With the knee flexed to 45 degrees and the leg externally rotated, a curved incision is made on the medial side of the knee. The position of this incision depends upon whether an anterior arthrotomy is required as well as an exploration of the popliteal fossa.

If both are to be exposed (Figure 3.15(a)), the incision should be about 15 cm in length, curving slightly forwards so that its apex lies approximately 2 cm medial to the patella. In this case the incision lies in front of the long saphenous vein.

If only the popliteal fossa is to be approached (Figure 3.15(b)) a curved incision is made of similar length, but well behind the medial border of the tibia below, curving backwards at the level of the knee joint along the line of semimembranosus above. In this case the incision lies behind the saphenous vein and nerve.

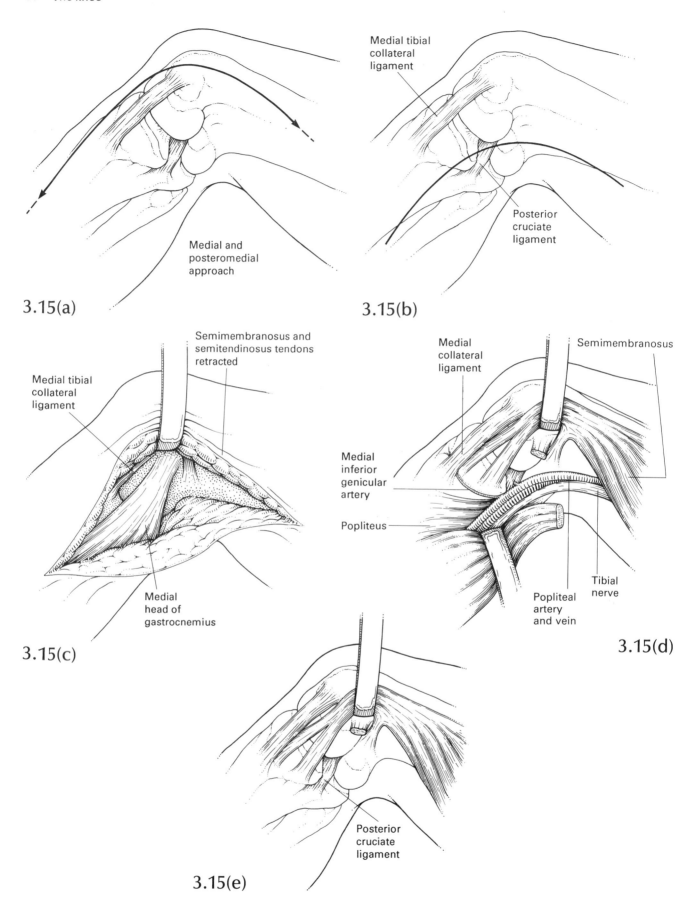

3.15(a)

Medial and posteromedial approach

3.15(b)

Medial tibial collateral ligament

Posterior cruciate ligament

3.15(c)

Medial tibial collateral ligament

Semimembranosus and semitendinosus tendons retracted

Medial head of gastrocnemius

3.15(d)

Medial collateral ligament

Semimembranosus

Medial inferior genicular artery

Popliteus

Popliteal artery and vein

Tibial nerve

3.15(e)

Posterior cruciate ligament

Approach

The incision is continued down to the deep fascia. If the anterior incision has been made a large flap of skin and subcutaneous tissue, containing the saphenous vein and nerve, must now be reflected posteriorly, exposing the superficial layer of the medial collateral ligament. In the case of the posterior incision, the deep fascia is incised in the line of the skin incision. Over the upper tibia the incision is deepened down to bone. A retractor is used to draw forward the tendons of semimembranosus and semitendinosus, exposing the posteromedial border of the tibia and the fascia covering the medial head of gastrocnemius. This fascia is incised and the muscle is traced upwards to its tendinous origin from the femur (Figure 3.15(c)). If access to the posterior cruciate ligament is required, the medial head of gastrocnemius is detached close to its origin (Figure 3.15(d),(e)).

Attention is now turned to the lower part of the wound where the popliteus muscle can be seen on the posterior surface of the upper tibia. The popliteus muscle is inserted into the medial side of the tibia at the oblique line at which can be seen the fibrous origin of soleus passing downwards and medially. At the upper border of popliteus the medial inferior genicular artery will be found running forwards, deep to the medial collateral ligament, just above its inferior attachment (Figure 3.15(d)).

The medial inferior genicular artery should be clamped, divided and ligated, the insertion of popliteus should be detached from the tibia and then the space between popliteus and the posterior capsule of the knee joint can be developed. It is safe to retract the popliteus muscle posteriorly since, together with popliteal fascia, it forms a pad which protects the medial popliteal nerve and the popliteal artery and vein. The middle genicular vessels, arising from the popliteal artery and vein, should now be ligated and divided with care as they are very short.

The posterior capsule of the knee joint can now be seen, together with the posterior cruciate ligament which arises extrasynovially from the posterior margin of the tibia (Figure 3.15(e)).

If the anterior curved incision has been used, it is possible at this stage to make an anterior arthrotomy into the knee and to inspect or repair the medial collateral ligament of the knee.

Indications

This approach can be used for the repair or reconstruction of the posterior cruciate ligament and for repairs of the posterior oblique ligament and the medial collateral ligament.

Lateral approach (Bruser)

Access

This approach affords good exposure of the lateral compartment of the knee joint without division of the fibular collateral ligament.

Approach

The knee is fully flexed so that the foot rests on the operating table. The incision is made at the level of, and parallel to, the joint line (Figure 3.16) from the patellar tendon in front to an imaginary line joining the head of the fibula to the lateral femoral condyle. The subcutaneous tissue is divided in the line of the incision to expose the iliotibial band whose fibres, with the knee in full flexion, also run in the line of the incision. The band is split in the line of its fibres at the level of the joint, taking care to avoid damage to the fibular collateral ligament which is relaxed in this position (Figure 3.16). The margins of the iliotibial band can now be retracted to expose the synovium of the knee and the lateral inferior genicular artery which lies between the collateral ligament and the synovium at the posterior aspect of the meniscus.

The synovium can now be incised to expose the lateral meniscus.

Indications

Complete exposure of the lateral meniscus for excision or repair.

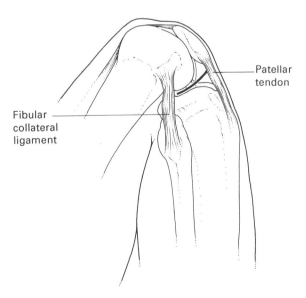

Patellar
tendon

Fibular
collateral
ligament

Lateral approach (Bruser)

3.16

Lateral approach to the distal femur (Rüedi, von Hochstetter and Schlumpf)

Access

This approach exposes the whole of the lower femoral shaft including the femoral condyles and can be extended by detaching the tibial tubercle to give wide access to the knee joint.

Incision

The skin is incised along a line joining the greater trochanter, the lateral femoral condyle and the tibial tuberosity (Figure 3.17).

Approach

The fascia lata is split in the line of the incision starting just in front of Gerdy's tubercle, continuing in a proximal direction in the line of the fibres (Figure 3.18). Vastus lateralis is detached from the intermuscular septum and from the femur. The superior lateral genicular artery is ligated and divided, as are the perforating vessels to vastus lateralis. The capsule of the knee joint is entered in the line of the incision just in front of the superior attachment of the lateral collateral ligament (Figure 3.19).

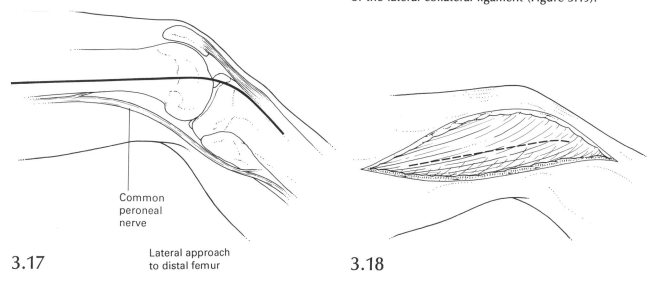

Common
peroneal
nerve

3.17   Lateral approach
to distal femur

3.18

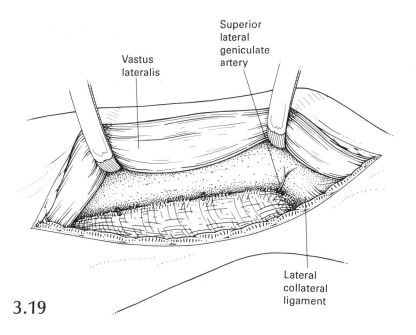

Vastus
lateralis

Superior
lateral
geniculate
artery

Lateral
collateral
ligament

3.19

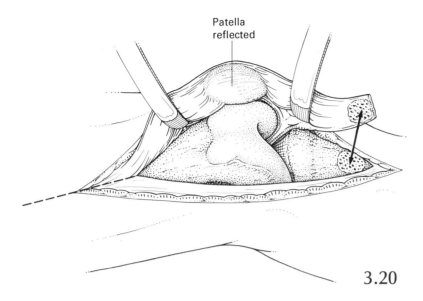

Patella
reflected

3.20

If further exposure is required the incision is continued distally, just lateral to the patellar tendon, as far as the lower limit of the tibial tuberosity which can then be detached with the patellar tendon. The patella is now mobilized superomedially dissecting the patellar tendon free from the infrapatellar fat pad (Figure 3.20).

Indications

This approach gives ideal exposure for the internal fixation of supracondylar and articular fractures of the femur. It may also be indicated for the treatment of tumours of the lower femoral shaft.

Lateral parapatellar approach to the knee and proximal tibia (Rüedi, von Hochstetter and Schlumpf)

Access

This approach provides limited access to the knee joint and to the lateral tibial condyle. It may be extended to expose most of the upper tibia, the knee joint and the femoral condyles by making a separate medial capsular incision after retracting the medial skin flap with the knee flexed.

Incision

The length of the incision depends on the access required and therefore a straight incision is preferred starting about 8 cm proximal to the patella over the distal insertion of vastus lateralis. It is continued distally along the lateral border of the patella and patellar tendon and ends just below the tibial tuberosity (Figure 3.21).

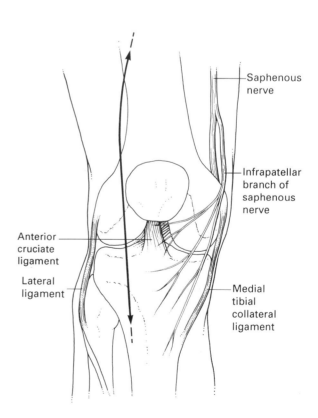

Saphenous nerve

Infrapatellar branch of saphenous nerve

Anterior cruciate ligament

Lateral ligament

Medial tibial collateral ligament

Lateral parapatellar approach

3.21

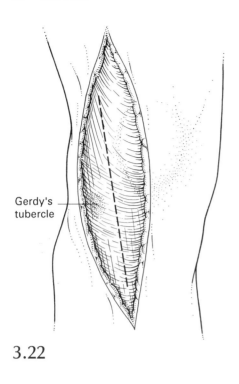

Gerdy's
tubercle

3.22

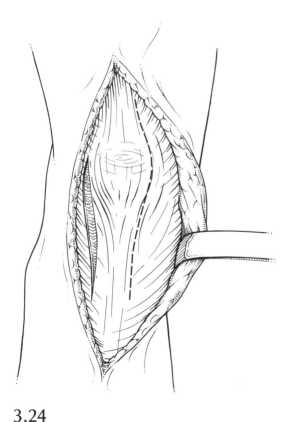

Tubercle
detached

3.23

3.24

Approach

The joint capsule is incised in the line of this incision
(Figure 3.22). Sharp dissection is continued laterally,
raising the lateral joint capsule, the iliotibial tract and the
extensor muscles from the tibia as a single sheet. It is an
advantage to detach Gerdy's tubercle with an osteotome.
The lateral dissection is continued posteriorly to the
lateral collateral ligament (Figure 3.23).

Note

At this stage it may be possible to treat fractures of the
lateral tibial plateau but if further exposure of the upper
tibia is required the skin flap should be dissected
medially, a medial parapatellar incision made into the joint
capsule and the patella then dislocated laterally (Figure
3.24). The medial capsule is freed from the upper tibia by
sharp dissection (Figure 3.25). If the proximal third of the
tibial shaft is to be exposed, the pes anserinus can be
detached, preferably with a thin shell of bone to facilitate
subsequent reattachment with a screw (Figure 3.26).

Indications

Fractures of the tibial condyles and proximal tibial shaft.
Cruciate ligament repair, medial collateral ligament repair
and tumours of the proximal tibia can all be dealt with by
this combined approach.

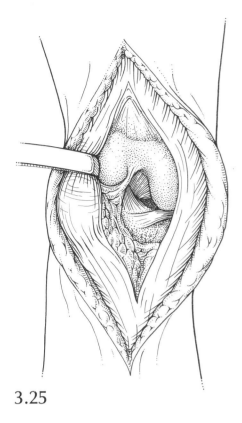

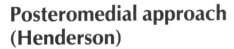

3.25

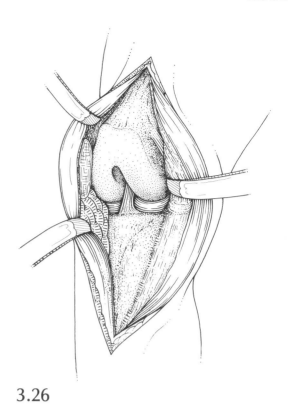

3.26

Posteromedial approach (Henderson)

Access

This exposure affords limited access to the posteromedial compartment of the knee.

Incision

With the knee flexed, a slightly curved incision is made from the adductor tubercle along the course of the posterior margin of the medial ligament and in front of the relaxed tendons of semimembranosus, semitendinosus, sartorius and gracilis muscles (Figure 3.27(a)).

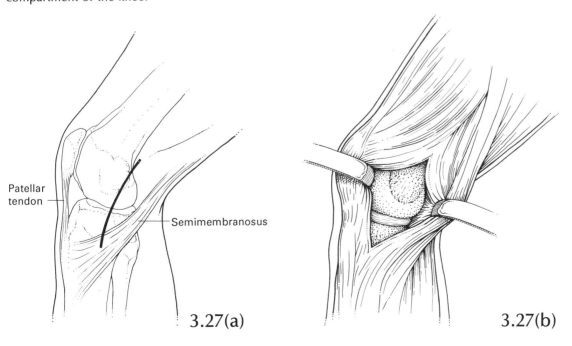

Patellar tendon

Semimembranosus

3.27(a)

3.27(b)

Approach

The oblique part of the tibial collateral ligament thus exposed is incised longitudinally and the capsule is opened in the same direction to enter the posteromedial compartment (Figure 3.27(b)).

Indications

Removal or repair of posterior horn of medial meniscus, removal of large loose bodies and drainage of the knee joint cavity.

Posterolateral approach (Henderson)

Access

This approach exposes the posterolateral aspect of the knee joint, the posterior third of the lateral meniscus and the lateral femoral condyle.

Incision

With the knee flexed, a curved incision is made on the lateral side of the knee, just in front of biceps femoris tendon and the head of the fibula (Figure 3.28(a)). The incision lies in front of the common peroneal nerve, which passes over the lateral aspect of the neck of the fibula.

Approach

Superiorly, the anterior aspect of the intermuscular septum is exposed down to its attachment to the linea aspera. The lateral femoral condyle and the origin of the fibular collateral ligament are exposed. The popliteus tendon, which lies between the biceps tendon and the fibular collateral ligament, is retracted posteriorly and a longitudinal incision through the capsule and synovium reveals the posterior compartment of the knee. Alternatively the lateral head of the gastrocnemius can be mobilized and retracted posteriorly. A vertical incision in the capsule will now expose the posterior part of the lateral compartment (Figure 3.28(b)).

Caution

The superior lateral genicular vessels may have to be coagulated or ligated as they pass across the lateral head of the gastrocnemius and the inferior lateral genicular vessels are vulnerable in the lower part of the wound as they pass forwards over popliteus to run deep to the lateral ligament anteriorly.

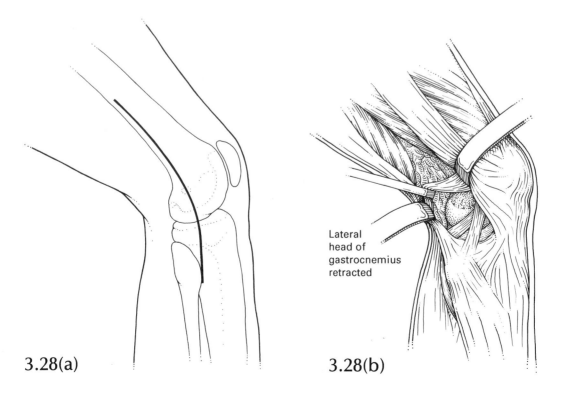

Lateral head of gastrocnemius retracted

3.28(a)　　　　3.28(b)

Indications

The removal of large loose bodies and posterolateral drainage of the knee joint cavity.

Skin incisions about the knee

Although the anatomy of the knee imposes certain limitations on the approaches to the joint, no such constraints have been imposed on the skin incisions and a very large number of incisions have been described, many of them eponymous. However, the healing of incisions over the knee is not universally satisfactory and some of the incisions have been abandoned by their authors after finding that there was a tendency for the skin margins to slough.

Not only do fashions change in surgery, but the patterns of disease change, so that many of the early approaches were designed merely to provide adequate drainage in cases of septic arthritis. Later, many different incisions were described to provide access for the removal of the menisci. Today, the emphasis has shifted towards approaches which provide access to several parts of the knee through the same incision, enabling surgeons to carry out the complicated procedures required for ligament reconstruction, necessitated both by contemporary aspirations and excesses in the field of sports.

MEDIAN PARAPATELLAR INCISIONS OF VON LANGENBECK AND PAYR

The median parapatellar incision of von Langenbeck (1878) and the so-called 'S' shape described by Payr (1917) have given rise to the anteromedial approach used today. The sharp curves in Payr's 'S' were not conducive to satisfactory wound healing, but the capsular incision probably resulted in less interference with the extensor mechanism. Langenbeck's gently curving skin incision has survived, together with Payr's capsular incision (Figure 3.29).

OBLIQUE PARAPATELLAR INCISION OF ERKES (Figure 3.30)

This incision follows the Langers lines over the knee. The slightly curved incision runs from the medial surface of the medial epicondyle of the femur to the insertion of the patellar tendon into the tibial tubercle. In order to permit displacement of the patella the fibres of origin of the vastus medialis are freed from the medial intermuscular septum. The advantage of this approach is said to be that the aponeurotic insertion of vastus medialis is not interfered with.

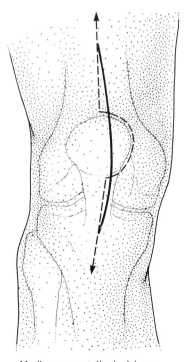

Median parapatellar incisions

3.29

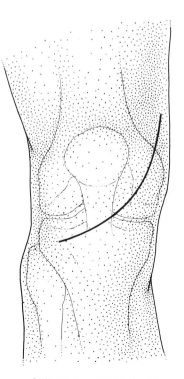

Oblique parapatellar incision

3.30

Incisions which interfere with the extensor mechanism

Although detachment of the tibial tubercle is described as an extension of the lateral approach to the distal femur (Rüedi, von Hochstetter and Schlumpf, 1984), as a general rule, approaches which involve division of the patella (either vertically or horizontally), or transection of either the patellar tendon or the tendon of the quadriceps muscle, are best avoided since they result in defective extensor function to a greater or lesser extent.

Putti (1917) described an inverted 'U' incision in which the quadriceps tendon was sectioned in the line of the incision or by various plastic incisions to facilitate lengthening of the tendon. Putti himself abandoned the incision because the skin did not always heal well (Figure 3.31).

Textor (1860) described a U-shaped incision which divided capsule and patellar tendon in line with the skin incision (Figure 3.31).

Ollier (1891) described an 'H' incision over the front of the knee.

None of the above incisions is recommended.

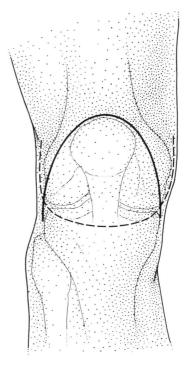

Incisions which interfere with the extensor mechanism

3.31

Incisions which divided the patella

Jones (1916) and Brackett and Hall (1917) used a curvilinear incision from 3 inches above the patella to the tibial tubercle. The quadriceps tendon, patella and patellar tendon were divided longitudinally at the junction of their medial and middle thirds, the patella being split with an osteotome or a saw.

Von Volkman (1977) advocated transverse section of the patella, whereas Devine (1931) described an approach which involved sagittal section of the patella.

These approaches are not recommended.

Similarly, the once popular so-called 'Mercedes' incision is now not recommended due to the problems of wound healing associated with it (Figure 3.32).

Incisions for meniscectomy

The various incisions for open meniscectomy are illustrated. With the advent of arthroscopic surgery they have become less relevant (Figures 3.33, 3.34).

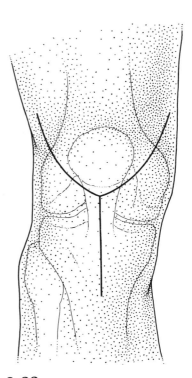

3.32

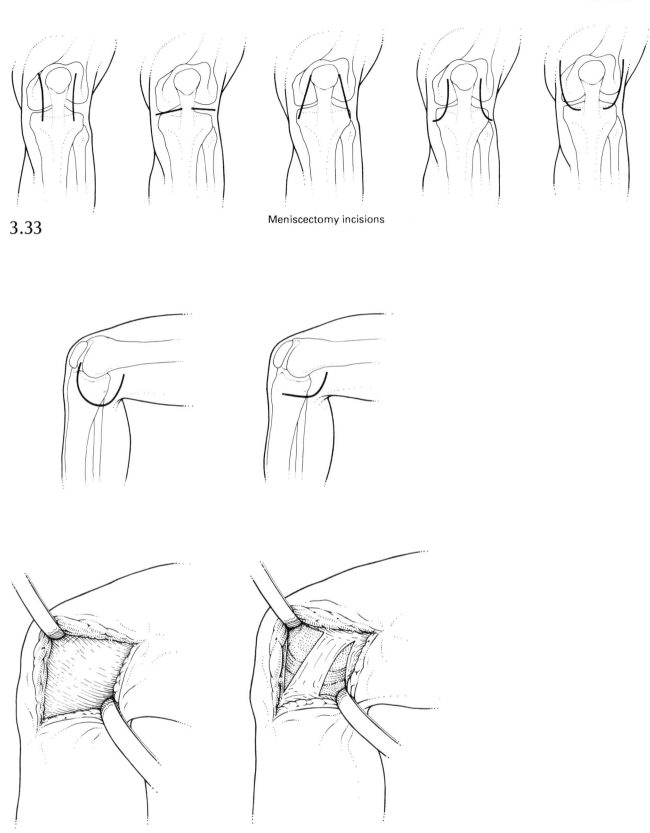

3.33

Meniscectomy incisions

Meniscectomy incisions
'not recommended'

3.34

Utility incisions

Utility incisions have come about through the need to expose several knee joint structures through one incision to facilitate the repair of complex ligamentous injuries. One such incision has already been described in relation to the medial and posteromedial approach (see p. 49). If the posterior compartment is not to be explored an S-shaped incision (Figure 3.35) can be employed to expose the medial ligament and to explore the front of the knee through an anterior capsular incision.

On the lateral side the choice of incision depends upon the structures to be exposed but in general the incision described in the lateral approach to the distal femur is the most useful (see p. 52).

More recently, McConnell (1976) has described a versatile incision which combines access to the anterior, posterior, medial and lateral sides of the knee with good cosmesis.

Incision (Figure 3.36)

With the knee fully flexed, the transverse anterior part of the incision is made by joining the medial flexion crease via the inferior pole of the patella to the lateral flexion crease. On the lateral side the incision is extended along the posterior margin of the iliotibial band as far proximally as necessary. On the medial side the incision is extended in a slightly posteromedial direction. Where possible, the fascia is incised in the line of the incision and raising flaps to expose the joint capsule is kept to a minimum to preserve the vascularity of the skin margins.

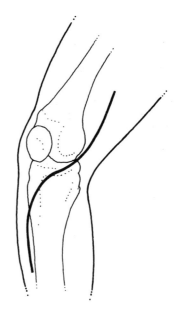

3.35

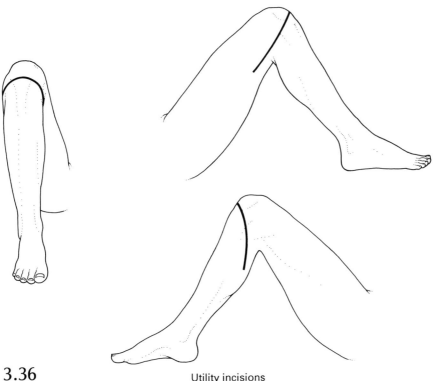

3.36   Utility incisions

References

Brackett, E. G. and Hall, C. L. (1917) Osteochondritis dissecans. *Am. J. Orthop. Surg.,* **XV**, 79

Brackett, E. G. and Osgood, R. B. (1911) The popliteal incision for the removal of joint mice in the posterior capsule of the knee joint. *Boston Med. Surg. J.,* **165**, 975

Bruser, D. M. (1960) A direct lateral approach to the lateral compartment of the knee joint. *J. Bone Joint Surg.,* **42B**, 3, 8

Devine, H. B. (1931) Exposure of the knee joint. *Br. J. Surg.,* **XIX**, 306

Erkes, F. (1929) Weitere Erfahrungen mit Physiologischer Schnitt Fuhrung zue Eroffnung des Kniegelenks. *Brunx Beitr. Klin. Chir.,* **CXLVII**, 221

Gillquist, J. and Hagberg, G. (1976) A new modification of the technique of arthroscopy of the knee joint. *Acta Chir. Scand.,* **142**, 123–130

Henderson, M. S. (1921) Posterolateral incision for the removal of loose bodies from the posterior compartment of the knee joint. *Surg. Gynecol. Obstet.,* **33**, 691

Insall, J. (1971) A mid-line approach to the knee. *J. Bone Joint Surg.,* **53A**, 1584

Jones, R. (1916) Disabilities of the knee joint. *Br. Med. J.,* **II**, 169

McConnell, J. C. (1976) A dynamic transpatellar approach to the knee. *South. Med. J.,* **69**, 567

Ollier, L. (1891) *Traite des Resections et des Opérations Conservatrices qu'on peut Practiquer sur le Systéme Osseux,* Masson et Cie, Paris

Payr, E. (1917) Einfaches und schonendes Verfahren zur beliebig Eroffnung des Kniegelenkes. *Zentralbl. Chir.,* **XLIV**, 921

Putti, V. (1917) La mobilizazione chirurgica delle anchilosi del ginocchio. *Chir. Organi. Mov.,* **1**, 1

Rüedi, T., von Hochstetter, A. and Schlumpf, R. (1984) *Surgical Approaches for Internal Fixation,* Springer, Berlin

Textor, K. (1860) Resection des Kniegelenkes. *Verh. Ges. Naturf. Arzte,* **XXXI**, 177

von Langenbeck, B. (1878) Zur Resection des Kniegelenkes. *Verh. Dtsch. Ges. Chir.,* **VII**, 34

von Volkman, R. (1977) Die Resection des Kniegelenkes mit Querer Durchsagung der Patella. *Dtsch. Med. Wohenschr.,* **III**, 389

Further reading

Abbott, L. C. and Carpenter, W. F. (1945) Surgical approaches to the knee joint. *J. Bone Joint Surg.,* **27**, 277

Chapter 4

The tibia and fibula

C. H. Rorabeck and J. R. Davey

RELEVANT ANATOMY – THE TIBIA

Superficial nerves

SUPERFICIAL PERONEAL NERVE

The superficial peroneal nerve is one of two terminal branches of the common peroneal nerve. After passing around the neck of the fibula, the common peroneal nerve pierces the deep fibres of the peroneus longus and divides into its superficial and deep branches. The superficial peroneal nerve descends in the substance of the peroneus longus until it reaches the proximal end of peroneus brevis and it then runs distally in the interval between extensor digitorum and peroneus brevis (anterior intermuscular septum). In the distal third of the leg, the nerve pierces the deep fascia and descends into the foot as two branches, the medial and intermediate dorsal cutaneous nerves of the foot.

SAPHENOUS NERVE

The saphenous nerve is the longest branch of the femoral nerve, arising in the femoral triangle and accompanying the femoral artery through the subsartorial canal to the adductor hiatus. It leaves the artery at this point and pierces the deep fascia at the posteromedial side of the knee, descending distally closely applied to the great saphenous vein. It crosses the distal third of the tibia in association with the great saphenous vein, and descends in front of the medial malleolus to end on the medial side of the foot.

SURAL NERVE

The sural nerve arises in the popliteal fossa as a terminal branch of the tibial nerve. It descends between the medial and lateral heads of gastrocnemius, just under the deep fascia which, in the proximal third of the calf, separates it from the short saphenous vein. Approximately half-way down the leg, the sural nerve pierces the deep fascia and accompanies the short saphenous vein to the back of the lateral malleolus. It supplies sensation to the lateral side of the foot and small toe.

Superficial veins

LONG SAPHENOUS VEIN

The long saphenous vein begins along the medial side of the foot and ascends in front of the medial malleolus, passing obliquely across the distal third of the medial border of the tibia. At the level of the knee it is found posteromedially.

SHORT SAPHENOUS VEIN

The short saphenous vein begins in the foot and runs behind the lateral malleolus, ascending the leg first lateral to the Achilles tendon and then in the mid-line of the gastrocnemius. As it ascends through the leg, it is superficial to the deep fascia until it reaches the popliteal space where it pierces the fascia to enter the popliteal vein. In the lower half of the leg it is accompanied by the sural nerve.

Deep nerves and vessels

ANTERIOR TIBIAL ARTERY AND DEEP PERONEAL NERVE

The anterior tibial artery arises as a terminal branch of the popliteal artery near the lower border of the popliteus muscle. There it passes forwards through a hiatus in the interosseous membrane and then descends distally on the front of the membrane. The deep peroneal nerve, arising as a terminal branch of the common peroneal nerve, pierces the anterior intermuscular septum and the substance of extensor digitorum longus to approach the anterior tibial artery from its lateral side. The anterior tibial artery and the deep peroneal nerve then descend together in the interval between tibialis anterior and extensor digitorum longus. They are initially deep in the leg, being applied closely to the interosseus membrane, but gradually become more superficial distally. Near the ankle joint they are crossed by the tendon of the extensor hallucis longus and enter the foot between extensor hallucis longus and extensor digitorum longus.

The anterior tibial artery gives off three named branches. The first, the anterior tibial recurrent, arises in the upper part of the front of the leg and accompanies the recurrent genicular nerve towards the knee. Injury to this vessel is unlikely through any of the usual approaches to the tibia. Distally in the leg, the anterior tibial artery gives off the lateral and medial malleolar branches. These may be injured through the anterior approach to the tibia, particularly if the incision is carried across the ankle joint.

The deep peroneal nerve continues to lie lateral to the artery in the leg and ends midway between the malleoli by dividing into lateral and medial terminal branches. In the leg, it gives motor branches to tibialis anterior, extensor hallucis longus, extensor digitorum longus and peroneus tertius. It also supplies extensor digitorum brevis through its lateral terminal branch.

POSTERIOR TIBIAL ARTERY AND TIBIAL NERVE

The posterior tibial artery, a branch of the popliteal artery, begins at the lower border of the popliteus muscle. The artery descends distally in the leg, covered by the soleus, and lying directly upon the fascia covering tibialis posterior, between it and the flexor hallucis longus. The tibial nerve, a terminal branch of the sciatic nerve, descends along with the posterior tibial artery. In the upper part of the leg both these structures lie on the posterior surface of popliteus, the nerve being medial to the artery, but then crossing behind the artery to run on its lateral side in the leg. In the middle of the leg, these two structures are found posteromedial to the tibialis posterior muscle and in the distal third of the leg they lie

between the Achilles tendon and the medial border of the tibia before passing behind the medial malleolus to enter the foot. The posterior tibial nerve gives motor branches to tibialis posterior as well as to flexor digitorum longus, flexor hallucis longus and soleus. Along with the posterior tibial artery, these structures may be injured through a posterolateral approach (Harmon) to the tibia if the surgeon fails to get deep to the tibialis posterior. The posterior tibial artery, in its distal third, gives off an anastomotic branch from its lateral side, which communicates directly with the peroneal artery. This branch is commonly divided during a posterolateral approach.

PERONEAL ARTERY

The peroneal artery arises from the posterior tibial artery approximately 2 or 3 cm below popliteus. The artery descends laterally crossing tibialis posterior, in front of the soleus to reach the fibula. It runs alongside the fibula distally on the interosseus membrane in front of flexor hallucis longus. Once again, injury to this artery is prone to occur through the posterolateral approach to the tibia, particularly in the middle and distal thirds.

SURGICAL APPROACHES TO THE TIBIA

- Anterior
- Medial
- Posterolateral (Harmon)
- Posterior (Banks and Laufman)

Anterior approach (Figure 4.1(a))

Access

The anterior approach to the tibia allows access to the lateral or medial border of the tibia. The incision affords excellent exposure for open reduction and internal fixation of fractures of the proximal, middle or distal thirds.

Incision

The skin incision begins 3 cm behind the crest of the tibia proximally (just behind Gerdy's tubercle) and extends distally in a straight line. The incision should not be placed directly over the crest of the tibia but rather 1.0 cm lateral to the crest of the tibia (Figure 4.1(b)). Distally the incision curves medially along the lateral edge of the tibialis anterior tendon. Great care should be taken in making this incision to ensure that the skin and subcutaneous tissues along with the deep fascia are incorporated in the flap.

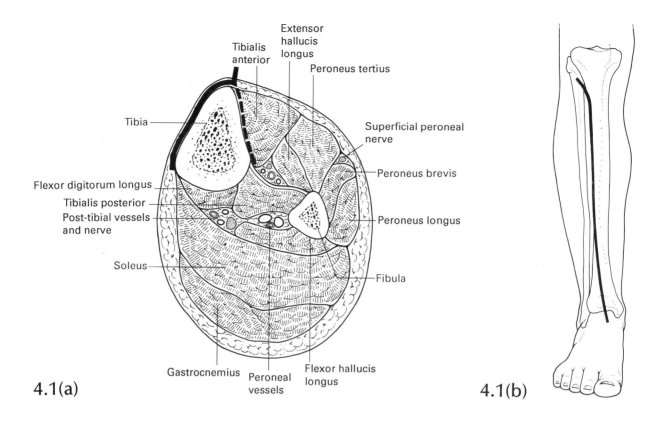

4.1(a)

4.1(b)

Approach

The skin and subcutaneous tissue are divided down to fascia, care being taken not to undermine the skin flap any more than is absolutely necessary in order to gain access to the subcutaneous anteromedial surface of the tibia.

To expose the lateral border of the middle four-fifths of the tibia, the fascia covering the anterior compartment muscle is detached from the crest of the tibia throughout the length of the incision (Figure 4.1(c)). Care should be taken in the depths of this incision to avoid injury to the anterior tibial artery and deep peroneal nerve. They are particularly prone to injury where they enter the anterior compartment in the extreme proximal limit of this approach.

Indications

For the exposure and internal fixation of fractures of the tibia.

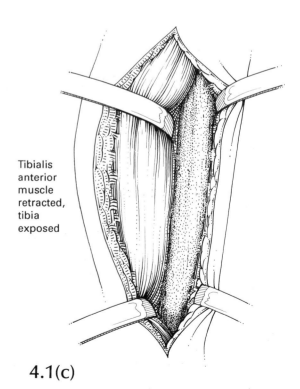

Tibialis anterior muscle retracted, tibia exposed

4.1(c)

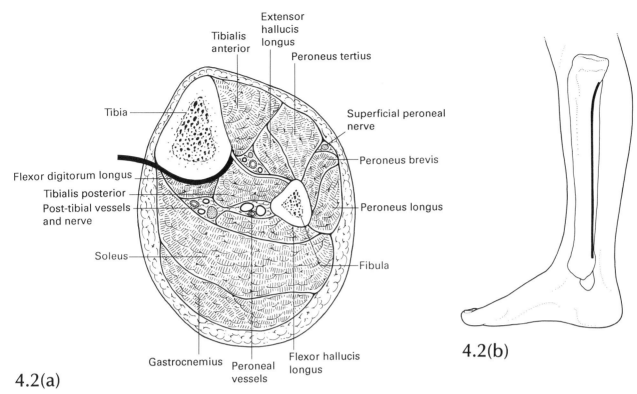

4.2(a)

4.2(b)

Medial approach (Figure 4.2(a))

Access

The medial approach to the tibia allows good access to the posterior border of the tibia.

Incision

The skin incision is straight, paralleling the posteromedial border of the tibia. The incision is placed 1.0 cm behind the posteromedial border of the tibia (Figure 4.2(b)) and great care should be taken to identify and protect the saphenous vein and nerve.

Approach

The periosteum overlying the posteromedial border of the tibia is now exposed and incised. Subperiosteal, or close extraperiosteal, dissection is carried out posteriorly to expose the entire posteromedial surface of the tibia (Figure 4.2(c)). In bone grafting procedures it is preferable to expose the posterior surface of the tibia by 'shingling' to raise a corticoperiosteal flap.

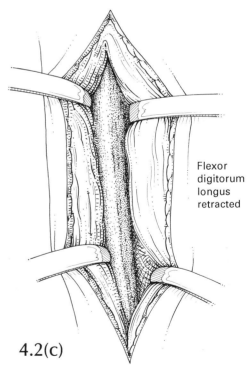

Flexor digitorum longus retracted

4.2(c)

Indications

This is useful for bone grafting procedures throughout the length of the bone, particularly in the proximal third. It is rarely used for the management of acute fractures, but is the preferred approach for autogenous grafting of non-unions in the proximal third of the tibia.

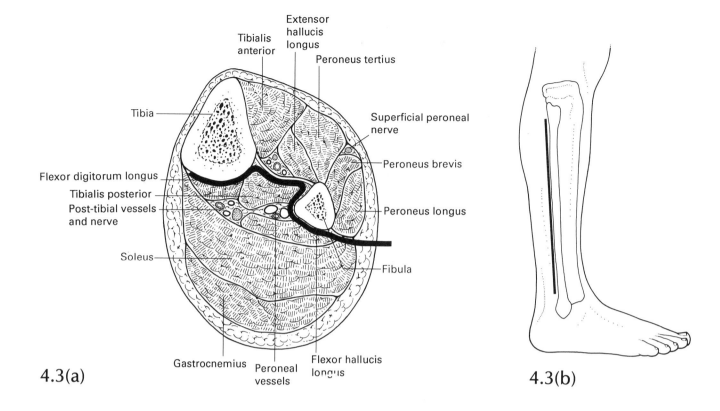

Tibialis anterior

Extensor hallucis longus

Peroneus tertius

Tibia

Superficial peroneal nerve

Peroneus brevis

Flexor digitorum longus

Tibialis posterior

Post-tibial vessels and nerve

Peroneus longus

Soleus

Fibula

Gastrocnemius   Peroneal vessels

Flexor hallucis longus

4.3(a)

4.3(b)

Posterolateral approach (Harmon) (Figure 4.3(a))

Access

This approach allows access to the posterior border of the tibia and the interosseus membrane.

Incision

The patient is positioned prone or in a lateral position with the affected leg prepared and draped free. The incision is planned as a straight line lying behind the shaft of the fibula extending in the interval between the peroneal tendons anteriorly and the gastrocnemius-soleus complex posteriorly (Figure 4.3(b)). Care must be taken distally to avoid damaging the sural nerve.

Approach

The interval between the peroneous longus and brevis anteriorly and the gastrocnemius and soleus posteriorly is identified and opened down to the fibula (Figure 4.3(c)).

Retraction in this interval will expose the muscle fibres of flexor hallucis longus, arising posterior to the fibula (Figure 4.3(c)).

The fibres of origin of flexor hallucis longus are detached to expose the posterior border of the fibula. Flexor hallucis longus is retracted posteriorly and medially with the gastrocnemius-soleus complex and peroneus longus and brevis are retracted anteriorly (Figure 4.3(d)).

The posterior surface of the shaft of the fibula is now exposed. By carefully staying subperiosteally along the posterior and medial border of the fibula and extending this dissection plane down onto the interosseus membrane, the fibres of origin of tibialis posterior can be detached from the interosseus membrane and retracted posteriorly to expose the posterior border of the tibia (Figure 4.3(e)).

The posterior tibial artery and vein lie between the tibialis posterior and flexor hallucis longus: they are not seen in this dissection but are protected by retracting tibialis posterior and flexor hallucis longus medially. Muscular branches of the peroneal artery are frequently encountered along with the peroneal artery in this incision and must be secured if divided.

Indications

This incision is useful for autogenous cancellous bone grafting of the distal half of the back of the tibia.

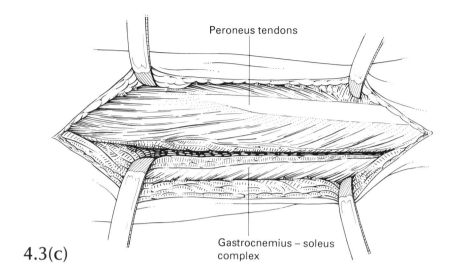

Peroneus tendons

Gastrocnemius – soleus
complex

4.3(c)

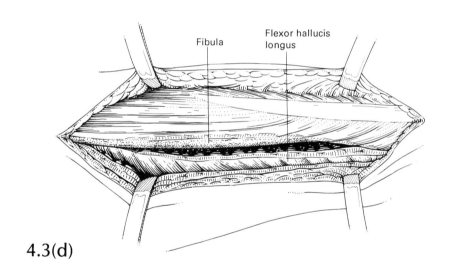

Fibula

Flexor hallucis
longus

4.3(d)

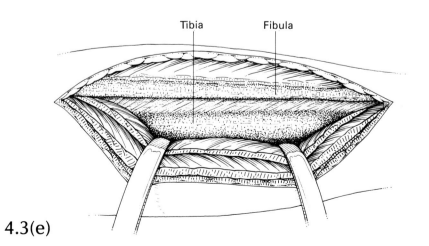

Tibia   Fibula

4.3(e)

Posterior approach to the superior medial region of the tibia (Banks and Laufman)

Access

This exposure affords access to the posterior surface of the proximal metaphyseal region of the tibia.

Incision

The patient is positioned prone and the incision is marked using the distal popliteal crease as a landmark and the medial border of the gastrocnemius-soleus complex as the other landmark. The incision follows the transverse popliteal crease and is then extended distally along the medial border of the calf (Figure 4.4(a)). Care must be taken to identify and protect terminal branches of the posterior cutaneous nerve of the thigh as well as terminal branches of the medial cutaneous nerve of the thigh, whenever possible.

Approach

Once the fascia is incised, the medial head of gastrocnemius is identified along with the lateral border of the semitendinosus muscle (Figure 4.4(b)). The semitendinosus is retracted medially and gastrocnemius is retracted laterally to expose the underlying popliteus muscle crossing the incision obliquely in its depth.

Flexor digitorum longus is also seen in the floor of the incision, distal to the popliteus muscle (Figure 4.4(c)). The interval between flexor digitorum longus and popliteus is identified and entered. Flexor digitorum longus is elevated subperiosteally from the posteromedial border of the back of the tibia and retracted distally, while popliteus is retracted proximally (Figure 4.4(d)).

One should not encounter the neurovascular bundle in this approach as it is applied to the deep surface of soleus. However, care must be taken in the retraction laterally of the gastrocnemius-soleus complex to avoid damage to these structures.

Indications

This is a useful approach to expose neoplastic lesions of the superomedial corner of the back of the tibia and may also be utilized to expose the posterior capsule and posterior cruciate region of the knee joint.

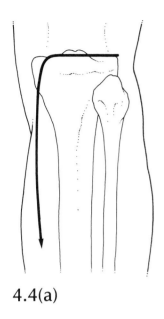

4.4(a)

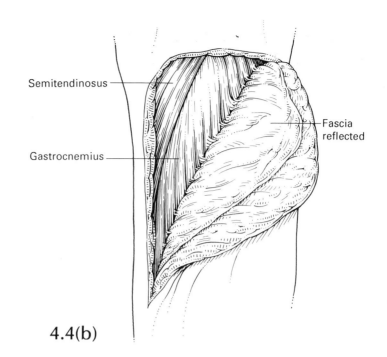

Semitendinosus

Gastrocnemius

Fascia
reflected

4.4(b)

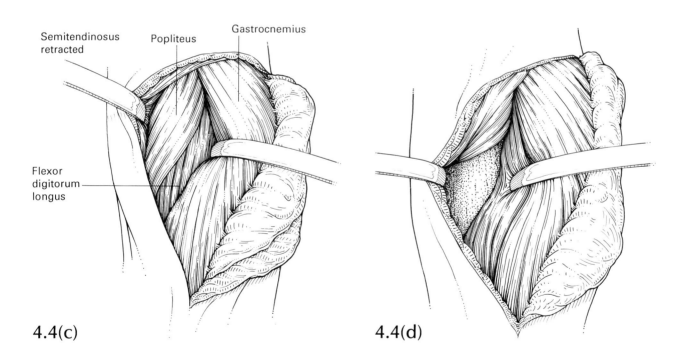

Semitendinosus
retracted

Popliteus

Gastrocnemius

Flexor
digitorum
longus

4.4(c)

4.4(d)

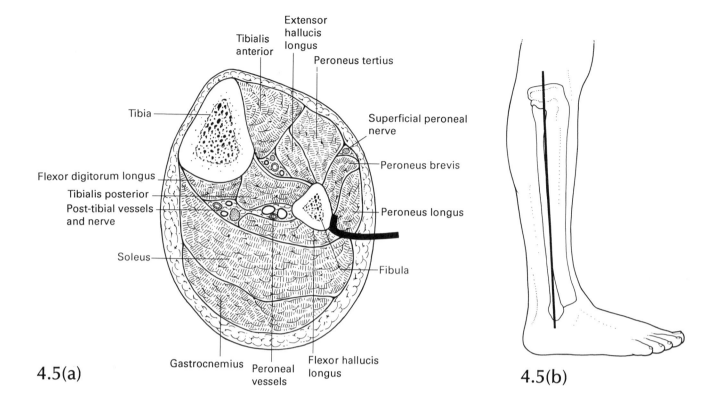

Tibialis
anterior

Extensor
hallucis
longus

Peroneus tertius

Superficial peroneal
nerve

Tibia

Peroneus brevis

Flexor digitorum longus

Tibialis posterior

Post-tibial vessels
and nerve

Peroneus longus

Soleus

Fibula

Gastrocnemius   Peroneal
vessels

Flexor hallucis
longus

4.5(a)

4.5(b)

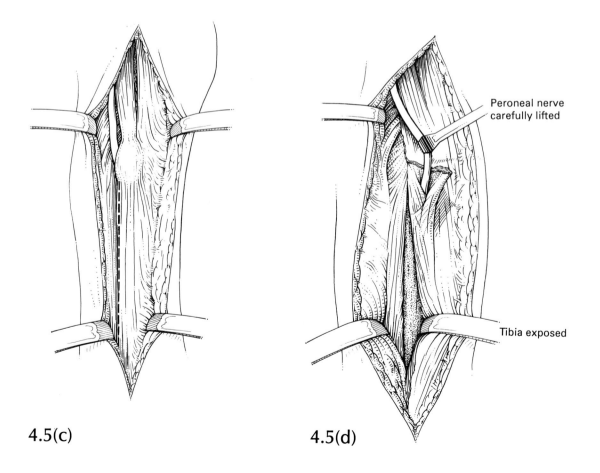

Peroneal nerve
carefully lifted

Tibia exposed

4.5(c)

4.5(d)

SURGICAL APPROACHES TO THE FIBULA

Posterolateral approach (Figure 4.5(a))

Access

The posterolateral approach to the fibula allows access to the entire shaft of the fibula; exposure of the proximal quarter can be difficult.

Incision

The patient is positioned in the straight lateral or prone position. The interval between the superficial posterior compartment and the lateral compartment is identified. The fibula is subcutaneous in its distal quarter and a straight incision is planned using these structures as landmarks (Figure 4.5(b)).

Approach

The interval is developed between the superficial post-erior compartment posteriorly and the peroneal muscles anteriorly. The incision is carried proximally and the peroneal nerve is isolated at the level of the posterior aspect of the biceps tendon (Figure 4.5(c)).

The nerve crosses the proximal end of the wound and enters the substance of peroneus longus. By isolating the nerve and by using gentle retraction, it can be carried anteriorly to expose the head of the fibula as necessary. The interval between the soleus posteriorly and the peroneal muscles anteriorly is now entered with the nerve safely out of the way and the dissection is carried down to expose the shaft of the tibia (Figure 4.5(d)).

Indications

This approach can be used for fibular osteotomy as a preliminary to tibial osteotomy. It is also useful for the harvesting of vascularized or free fibular bone grafts, and for the surgery of painful fibular non-union.

References

Banks, S. W. and Laufman, H. (1953) *An Atlas of Surgical Exposures of the Extremities,* W. B. Saunders, Philadelphia
Harmon, P. H. (1945) A simplified surgical approach to the tibia for bone grafting and fibular transference. *J. Bone Joint Surg.,* **27,** 496

Further reading

Kaplan, E. B. (1946) Posterior approach to the superolateral region of the tibia. *J. Bone Joint Surg.,* **28,** 805

Chapter 5

The ankle

C. L. Colton

RELEVANT ANATOMY

Superficial cutaneous nerves

Skin incisions around the ankle are planned to avoid the cutaneous nerves, wherever possible, as so many areas of bone are immediately deep to the skin that the formation of a neuroma can result in painful disability from footwear pressure.

SAPHENOUS NERVE

This nerve enters the ankle region, together with the long saphenous vein, along the line of the posteromedial border of the tibia, curving forwards to cross the ankle joint level just anterior to the medial malleolus. It then divides into numerous small branches to supply an area on the dorsomedial aspect of the tarsus (Figure 5.1).

SUPERFICIAL PERONEAL NERVE

Arising at the bifurcation of the common peroneal nerve in the upper third of the leg, the superficial peroneal nerve (formerly the musculocutaneous nerve) gives branches to the peroneal muscles and then emerges through the deep fascia of the leg between the peronei and the extensor digitorum longus. It then divides, above the ankle, into the medial and intermediate dorsal cutaneous nerves of the foot (Figure 5.2). The former crosses the ankle joint just lateral to the mid-line and then

divides into two branches which supply the medial aspect of the hallux and the adjacent sides of the second and third toes. The intermediate branch crosses the ankle over the front of the inferior tibiofibular joint and supplies the adjacent sides of the third, fourth and fifth toes.

SURAL NERVE (Figure 5.2(b))

After taking origin from the tibial nerve (formerly the medial popliteal nerve) and emerging from between the heads of gastrocnemius, the sural nerve pierces the deep fascia of the leg at the lateral edge of the Achilles tendon and descends to the interval between the lateral malleolus and the heel. From there it curves below the malleolar tip to run along the lateral border of the foot as far as the fifth toe.

Deep nerves and vessels

POSTERIOR TIBIAL NEUROVASCULAR BUNDLE (Figure 5.3)

This large bundle passes down to the ankle region from the posterior compartment of the leg, running behind the medial malleolus to enter the deep layers of the medial plantar structures. It lies on the posteromedial aspect of the distal tibial metaphyseal region between the tendons of flexor digitorum longus medially and of flexor hallucis longus on its lateral side. The nerve usually lies lateral to the vessels. The bundle, together with the tendons, is tightly bound down by a thickening of the deep fascia

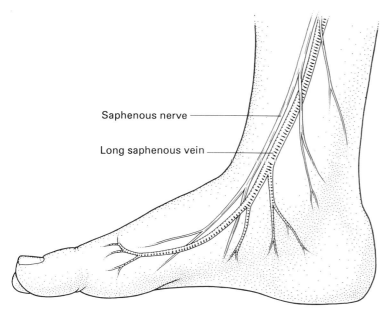

Saphenous nerve

Long saphenous vein

Superficial cutaneous nerves

5.1

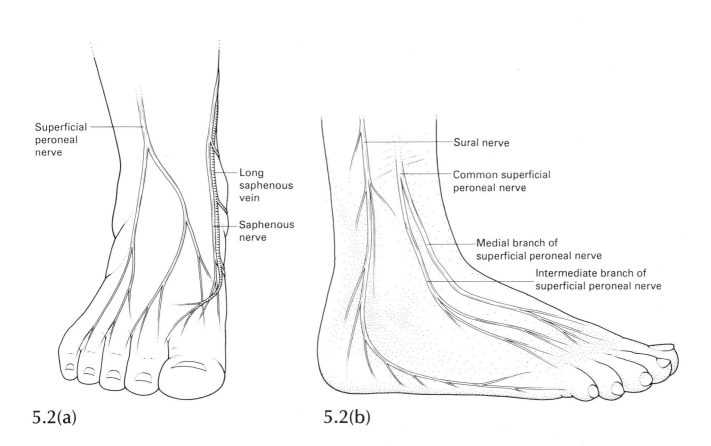

Superficial peroneal nerve

Long saphenous vein

Saphenous nerve

5.2(a)

Sural nerve

Common superficial peroneal nerve

Medial branch of superficial peroneal nerve

Intermediate branch of superficial peroneal nerve

5.2(b)

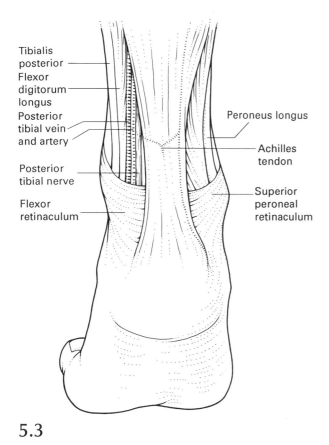

Tibialis posterior

Flexor digitorum longus

Posterior tibial vein and artery

Posterior tibial nerve

Flexor retinaculum

Peroneus longus

Achilles tendon

Superior peroneal retinaculum

5.3

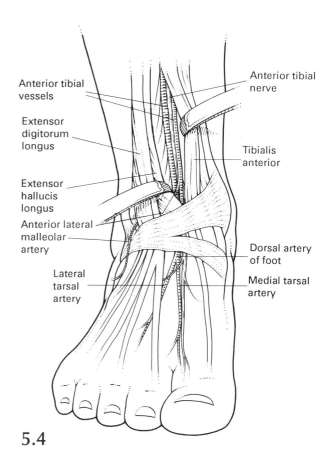

Anterior tibial vessels

Extensor digitorum longus

Extensor hallucis longus

Anterior lateral malleolar artery

Lateral tarsal artery

Anterior tibial nerve

Tibialis anterior

Dorsal artery of foot

Medial tarsal artery

5.4

which requires careful dissection if they are to be explored and mobilized. Just above the level of the ankle joint the artery sometimes gives a laterally running branch which communicates with the peroneal artery.

PERONEAL ARTERY

This vessel, of greatly variable size, arises from the posterior tibial artery, usually in the middle third of the leg, and passes distally along the interosseous membrane, adjacent to the fibula, between the tibialis posterior and the flexor hallucis longus muscles (occasionally within the latter's substance). It then crosses over the back of the inferior tibiofibular syndesmosis, deep to the flexor hallucis longus, and supplies branches to the lateral and posterior aspects of the heel.

ANTERIOR TIBIAL NEUROVASCULAR BUNDLE (Figure 5.4)

The anterior tibial artery, nerve and vein (from medial to lateral) pass deep to the extensor retinaculum over the front of the ankle, lying between the tendons of tibialis anterior and extensor hallucis longus in the proximal part of its course, and then between the tendons of extensor hallucis longus and extensor digitorum longus more distally. The tendon of the long extensor of the big toe

crosses the bundle superficially from lateral to medial at about the ankle joint level. At this level the artery gives off a virtually horizontal, laterally running branch – the anterior lateral malleolar artery. Apart from the tether provided by this vessel and by small venous branches communicating medially with the long saphenous vein, the bundle is relatively mobile on the underlying bone and joint capsule. The bundle then continues into the foot running towards the base of the second metatarsal, the artery becoming the dorsalis pedis vessel. Just below the level of the joint, the bundle gives rise to the lateral tarsal vessels and to the laterally coursing motor nerve to extensor digitorum brevis.

Ligaments

LATERAL LIGAMENT COMPLEX (Figure 5.5)

The lateral ligament complex of the ankle consists of three main fasciculi:

1. Anterior talofibular ligament.
2. Calcaneofibular ligament.
3. Posterior talofibular ligament.

The anterior talofibular ligament is a condensation of the ankle joint capsule arising from the anterior border of the

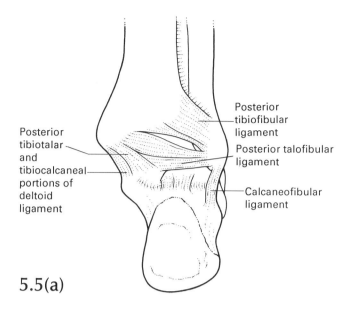

5.5(a)

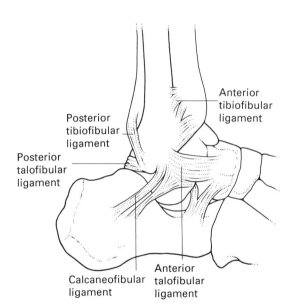

5.5(b)

lateral malleolus and taking a short course to be inserted into the lateral aspect of the talar neck between the articular surfaces of the ankle and the talonavicular joints. It is always the first structure to be torn in disruptions of the lateral ligament complex (Glasgow, Jackson and Jamieson, 1980).

The calcaneofibular fasciculus is a strong, discreet, ligamentous band taking origin from the tip of the lateral malleolus and running backwards, almost horizontally, to insert into the superolateral surface of the body of the os calcis. The superficial surface of this ligament is integral with the floor of the peroneal sheath.

The posterior talofibular ligament arises from just behind the tip of the lateral malleolus to be attached to the posterior tubercle of the talus.

DELTOID LIGAMENT

As its name suggests, this is a triangular ligament, of great strength, providing the medial tether of the tibiotalar articulation. It arises from the tip and medial face of the medial malleolus and fans out to an almost linear insertion along the medial aspect of the talus, immediately above the lower edge of the medial articular facet of that bone. These fibres constitute the tough, deep portion of the deltoid ligament and are relatively short. A broader, more superficial layer inserts more widely into the navicular, the sustentaculum tali, the medial tubercle of the posterior process of the talus and into the intervening capsular fibres.

SURGICAL APPROACHES

- Anterolateral (Campbell, 1949)
- Anteromedial
- Posterolateral
- Posteromedial
- Posterior
- Transfibular (Gatellier and Chastang, 1924)
- Medial transmalleolar (König and Schafer, 1929)

Anterolateral approach (Campbell)

Positioning

The patient is positioned supine on the operating table with a foam pad beneath the drapes to support the ankle. A 'sand-bag' beneath the ipsilateral buttock improves access.

Access

This exposure affords access to the anterior surface of the distal tibia as far medially as the anterior lip of the medial malleolus and laterally to the anterior and lateral faces of the distal fibula, together with the anterior talofibular ligament (Figure 5.6).

Incision (Figure 5.7)

A longitudinal incision is made starting approximately 7 cm above the ankle joint, 1 cm lateral to the anterior

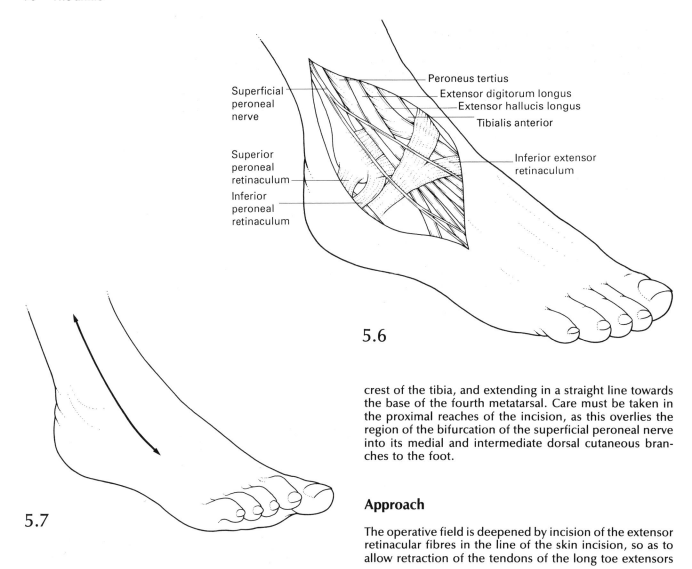

Superficial peroneal nerve

Superior peroneal retinaculum

Inferior peroneal retinaculum

Peroneus tertius
Extensor digitorum longus
Extensor hallucis longus
Tibialis anterior
Inferior extensor retinaculum

5.6

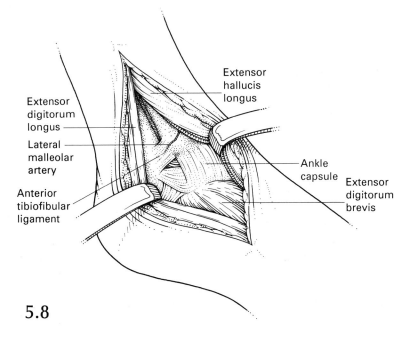

5.7

crest of the tibia, and extending in a straight line towards the base of the fourth metatarsal. Care must be taken in the proximal reaches of the incision, as this overlies the region of the bifurcation of the superficial peroneal nerve into its medial and intermediate dorsal cutaneous branches to the foot.

Approach

The operative field is deepened by incision of the extensor retinacular fibres in the line of the skin incision, so as to allow retraction of the tendons of the long toe extensors

Extensor digitorum longus

Lateral malleolar artery

Anterior tibiofibular ligament

Extensor hallucis longus

Ankle capsule

Extensor digitorum brevis

5.8

medially and that of peroneus tertius laterally. This then exposes the anterior capsule of the ankle joint, on the surface of which may be seen the anterior lateral malleolar vessels (Figure 5.8). The ankle joint may be entered by capsular incision, horizontal or vertical according to the requirements of the particular procedure.

To reach the lateral face of the fibula it may be necessary to mobilize the tendon of peroneus tertius medially, but the access here is somewhat limited (Figure 5.9). The full extent of the medial access afforded by this exposure is obtained by mobilization and medial retraction of the tendons of the long digital extensors and the anterior neurovascular bundle, which can be slackened by dorsiflexing the foot (Figure 5.10). Distal extension of this approach is by elevation of the belly of extensor digitorum brevis and its retraction medially. This permits exposure of the sinus tarsi and subtalar joint laterally and of the talar neck and talonavicular joint medially (Figure 5.11). During this extension, the lateral tarsal vessels cross the field and may require division. The width of this exposure is considerable and it has been nicknamed the 'universal incision' for the foot and ankle – a sacrifice of truth to hyperbole!

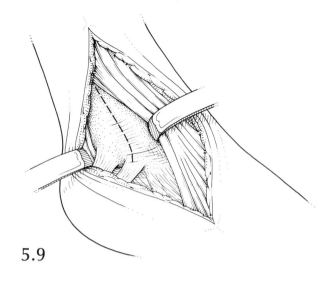

5.9

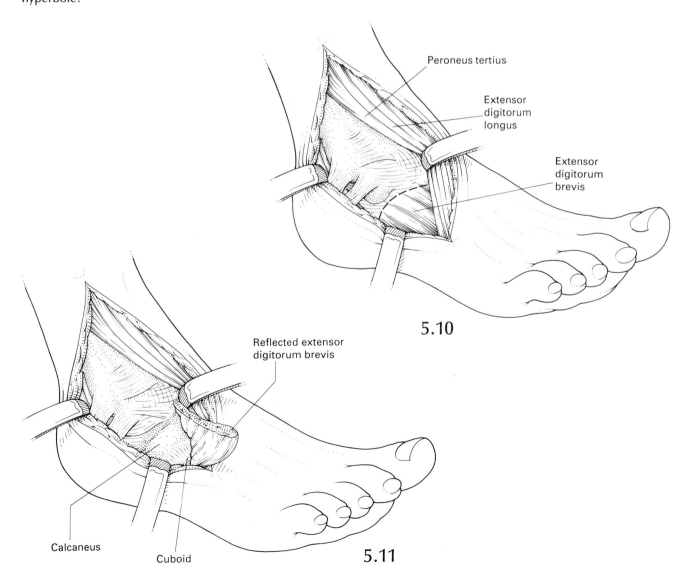

Peroneus tertius

Extensor digitorum longus

Extensor digitorum brevis

5.10

Reflected extensor digitorum brevis

Calcaneus

Cuboid

5.11

Indications

The anterolateral approach is used for anterolateral marginal fractures of the tibia, not involving the medial malleolus, associated fractures of the lateral malleolus and in anterolateral dislocation of the talus. It gives excellent access to the anterior talofibular ligament, the anterior syndesmosis and lesions of the front of the ankle. It may also be used for surgery in the region of the sinus tarsi and even for astragalectomy.

Anteromedial approach

Positioning

The patient is positioned supine on the operating table with a foam pad beneath the drapes to support the ankle. A 'sand-bag' beneath the opposite buttock is helpful.

Access

The anteromedial approach affords access to the whole of the front of the distal tibia and ankle joint, the medial malleolus and the anterior tibial tubercle (of Tillaux).

Incision (Figure 5.12(a))

The proximal portion of the skin incision is, in fact, a distal extension of the anterior incision for the exposure of the tibial shaft, 1 cm lateral to the anterior crest of the tibia, running parallel to it and then, over the distal quarter of the tibia, curving gently medially to midway between the tip of the medial malleolus and the navicular tubercle.

Approach (Figure 5.12(b))

This skin incision crosses the path of the long saphenous vein and saphenous nerve and if wide exposure is desired, division of these structures may be inevitable, although the nerve should be preserved whenever possible. The dissection is deepened to periosteum along the medial border of the tibialis anterior tendon, which, along with the long extensor tendons and the neurovascular bundle, can be freed on their deep surfaces and retracted laterally with the foot dorsiflexed (Figure 5.13). By this manoeuvre it is possible to reach as far lateral as the anterior tibial tubercle, but if liberal access to that region is required then a separate dissection between the extensor hallucis longus tendon and the neurovascular bundle medially and the long toe extensors laterally will improve this exposure (Figure 5.14).

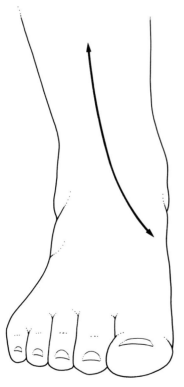

5.12(a)

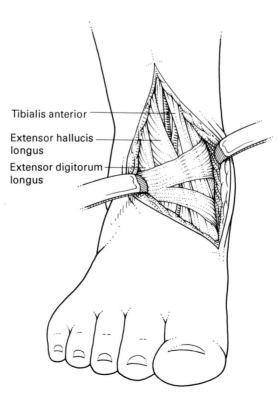

Tibialis anterior

Extensor hallucis longus

Extensor digitorum longus

5.12(b)

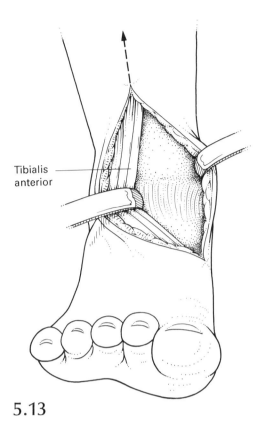

Tibialis
anterior

5.13

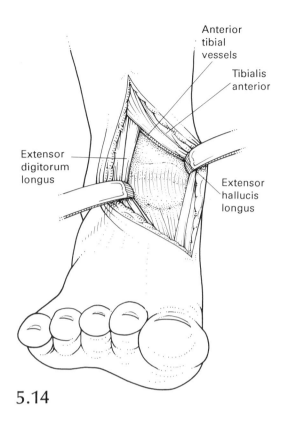

Anterior
tibial
vessels

Tibialis
anterior

Extensor
digitorum
longus

Extensor
hallucis
longus

5.14

Indications

This approach is widely regarded as the one of choice for compression fractures of the distal tibia ('pilon' fractures) and supramalleolar tibial fractures, as well as for fractures of the tibial shaft extending down into the ankle. Lesions of the anterior regions of the distal tibia and of the ankle joint are easily reached by this method.

Posterolateral approach

Positioning

The patient is positioned supine with a large 'sand-bag' under the ipsilateral buttock to tilt the leg into internal rotation.

This can be combined with the posteromedial approach by using the '4' posture to gain access to the inner side (Figure 5.15).

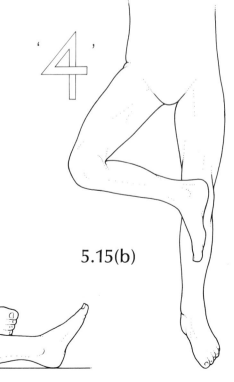

'4'

5.15(b)

5.15(a)

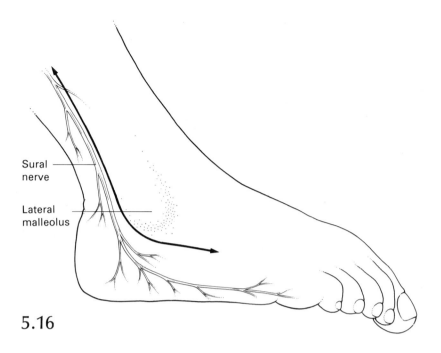

5.16

Access

This approach permits exposure of the distal fibular shaft and the lateral malleolus, extending forwards to give access to the anterior aspect of the inferior tibiofibular syndesmosis and posteriorly to gain the posterolateral quadrant of the distal tibia.

Incision (Figure 5.16)

The skin incision skirts the posterior border of the lower third of the fibula, anterior to the line of the sural nerve.

Below the level of the tip of the lateral malleolus it curves, in a 'hockey stick' fashion, forwards to the region of the peroneal tubercle. In this lower curved portion the sural nerve is vulnerable and must be carefully sought and protected.

Approach

Incision of the subcutaneous fascia overlying the lateral surface of the fibula permits blunt dissection to proceed anteriorly, exposing the anterior inferior tibiofibular ligament and anterior tibial tubercle. Similar dissection

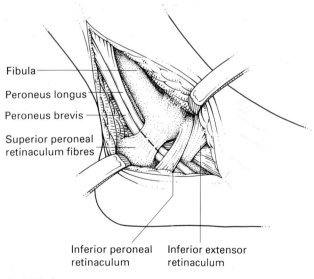

5.17(a)

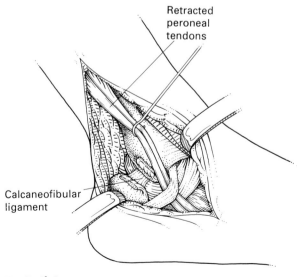

5.17(b)

beneath the posterior edge of the wound exposes the sheath and retinaculum of the peroneus longus and brevis tendons. Incision of this sheath and the retinacular fibres allows mobilization of the tendons forwards. Great care must be taken to preserve the cut retinacular fibres so that they may be repaired during closure to prevent recurrent anterior subluxation of the tendons (Figure 5.17(a)). This then exposes the posterior border of the fibula and, at the level of the malleolus, the surface of the posterior talofibular ligament can be followed by blunt dissection to lead to the posterior process of the talus (Figure 5.17(b)). From this point, blunt dissection can be carried proximally to gain the posterior surface of the tibia. It is during this stage of the approach that the peroneal artery is likely to be encountered; unless it is recognized and secured, it can be damaged, causing troublesome bleeding. At the ankle level, the fibula is on a more posterior plane than the posterior aspect of the distal tibia and this postero-lateral dissection is deeper and more difficult than the inexperienced operator may initially expect. For this reason, a long incision is advisable in order to avoid forceful soft tissue retraction.

Indications

The posterolateral approach is the exposure of choice for the fixation of fractures of the distal fibula and of the lateral malleolus, especially where an associated posterior lip fracture of the tibia (Volkmann's fracture) is judged to be more posterolateral than posteromedial. It is also ideally suited for procedures on the peroneal tendons, in particular some reconstructive operations for lateral instability of the ankle (Evans, 1953; Gordes and Vern-stein, 1980). The plantaris graft procedures of Sefton *et al.* (1979) and Marti *et al.* (1976) are, however, better undertaken through the anterolateral approach.

Posteromedial approach

Positioning

The supine position is adopted but the knee is flexed, the hip externally rotated and the ankle laid on the shin of the other leg, suitably padded with a small pillow beneath the drapes – the '4' position (Figure 5.15).

Access

This approach is capable of exposing the whole of the medial malleolus and the medial and posteromedial aspects of the distal tibia. It also affords access to the tendons and neurovascular bundle behind the distal medial tibia.

Incision (Figure 5.18)

The proximal starting point of the incision depends on the extent of access required. Only the lower portion of the incision will be utilized for limited exposure of, say, isolated fractures of the medial malleolus. The incision begins at the chosen level and runs distally, parallel to and 1 cm behind the posteromedial border of the tibia, curving anteriorly below the medial malleolus to the navicular tubercle.

Approach

Deepening the incision through the subcutaneous fat and fascia reveals the deep fascia over the tendons of tibialis posterior and flexor digitorum longus, the posterior tibial neurovascular bundle and both tendon and belly ('beef to the heel') of flexor hallucis longus (Figure 5.19). Blunt dissection forwards on the surface of this fascia leads to its anterior attachment to the posteromedial border of the tibia proximally and to the medial malleolus distally. In this latter region, it is thickened to form the flexor retinaculum. For access to the posteromedial quadrant of the distal tibia, it is necessary very carefully to open the deep fascia from above distally, in the line of the incision, and to expose the tendons and neurovascular bundle behind the tibia and medial malleolus (Figure 5.20), prior to establishing a plane of dissection between the bundle medially and flexor hallucis laterally. This is aided by plantarflexion of the foot to slacken these posterior structures. At, or just above, the ankle, the posterior tibial artery occasionally gives off a laterally running communi-cating branch (to the peroneal artery) which must be sought and secured.

Indications

The posteromedial approach is suitable for the fixation of fractures of the medial malleolus (unless they extend well into the anterior lip of the tibia, when the anteromedial

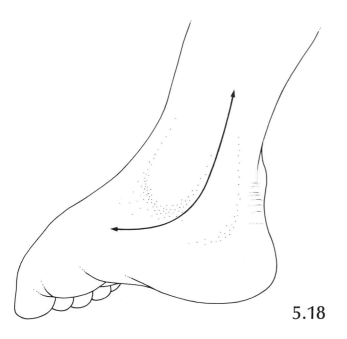

5.18

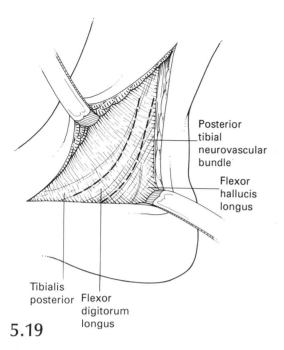

Posterior tibial neurovascular bundle

Flexor hallucis longus

Tibialis posterior   Flexor digitorum longus

5.19

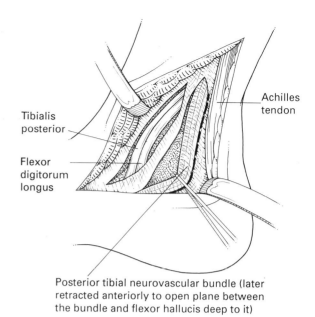

Achilles tendon

Tibialis posterior

Flexor digitorum longus

Posterior tibial neurovascular bundle (later retracted anteriorly to open plane between the bundle and flexor hallucis deep to it)

5.20

approach is more appropriate) and of the posterior 'malleolus' of the tibia (Volkmann's fracture) where this fragment is judged to be more posteromedial than posterolateral. It also affords access for exploration of the tendons and neurovascular bundle behind the medial malleolus.

Posterior approach

Positioning

The patient is laid prone on the operating table with a shaped foam wedge support beneath the drapes (Figure 5.21).

Access

The posterior approach gives excellent access to the back of the distal tibia, the posterior process of the talus and the superior aspect of the body of the os calcis. The lateral limit of the exposure is the inferior tibiofibular joint and, medially, access beyond the posterior lip of the medial malleolus is not practical.

Incision (Figure 5.22)

A straight mid-line ('stocking seam') skin incision is made over the length of the Achilles tendon, exposing its paratenon and its insertion into the heel.

Approach

A long, oblique or 'Z' division of the Achilles tendon is made and the ends, wrapped in moistened swabs, are retracted up and down (Figure 5.23(a)). The layer of deep fascia over the fat pad behind the ankle is incised and the fat pad removed. This exposes the interval between the flexor hallucis longus medially and, laterally, the peroneal muscles. This interval is then developed to expose the back of the tibia and ankle, the posterior tubercle of the talus and, if required, the upper surface of the body of the os calcis (Figure 5.23(b)). Care should be taken to recognize the peroneal artery in the lateral extent of the exposure and also any communicating vessels running horizontally across the back of the ankle capsule. It is better to divide these formally, if necessary, rather than to have to deal with their bleeding at a later stage (which may be after recovery from anaesthesia if a tourniquet has been used!). The Achilles tendon is carefully repaired during closure of the wound.

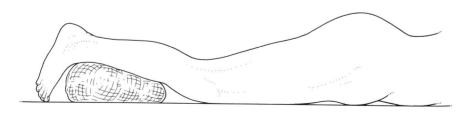

5.21

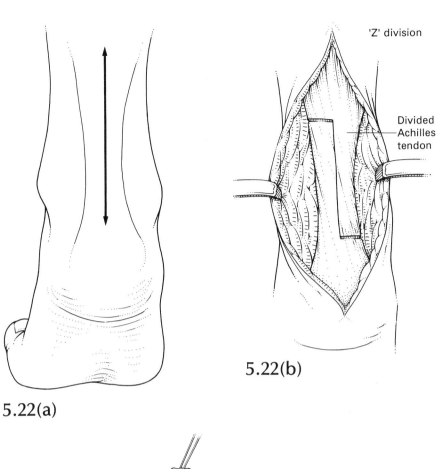

'Z' division

Divided
Achilles
tendon

5.22(b)

5.22(a)

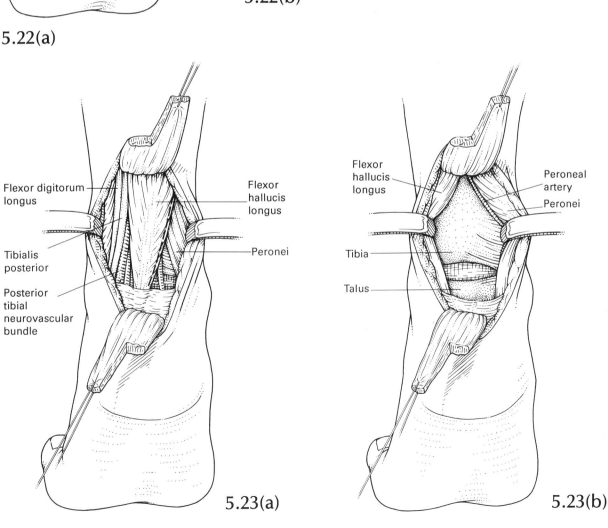

Flexor digitorum
longus

Flexor
hallucis
longus

Tibialis
posterior

Peronei

Posterior
tibial
neurovascular
bundle

5.23(a)

Flexor
hallucis
longus

Peroneal
artery

Peronei

Tibia

Talus

5.23(b)

Indications

This exposure is not commonly used for fractures, although difficult reconstruction of the posterior tibia is better undertaken by this direct approach than from posteromedially or posterolaterally. White (1974) and Colton (1982) have recommended its use for posterior arthrodesis of the ankle. It is certainly valuable for the exploration of lesions of bone or joint in the zone of access (see above).

Transfibular approach (Gatellier and Chastang)

Positioning

The patient is positioned supine on the operating table with a foam pad beneath the drapes to support the ankle. A 'sand-bag' beneath the ipsilateral buttock improves lateral access.

Access

The transfibular approach can be used to gain access to the lateral portion of the ankle joint and to the incisura fibularis.

Incision

This is as for the posterolateral approach (see p. 79).

Approach (Figure 5.24)

The principle of the approach rests upon making an osteotomy of the fibular shaft and turning down the distal portion, hinging distally on the lateral ligament complex. At about 7.5 cm above the ankle, an oblique hole is drilled upwards and medially in the coronal plane through the fibula and then an oblique fibular osteotomy is made in a plane perpendicular to the drill hole axis and in the sagittal plane, so that the hole passes through the centre of the cut bony surface (Figure 5.24(a),(b)). The lateral half of this hole is then over-drilled to allow later fixation with a lag screw through a fibular plate (Figure 5.24(c)).

The distal fibular fragment is freed by mobilization of the peronei from it and careful division of the ligaments of the inferior tibiofibular syndesmosis. This should then permit the fibula to be turned down on its lateral ligament, thus exposing the lateral facet of the talus and the lateral surface of the distal tibia (Figure 5.24(d)).

Repair is by suture of the ligaments of the syndesmosis after fixation of the fibular osteotomy as above.

Indications

This approach is not commonly used and was devised by Gatellier and Chastang (1924) for the fixation of large posteromedial fractures of the posterior tibial 'malleolus'. It is, however, a fairly extensive and disruptive dissection and alternative approaches, if appropriate, are to be preferred. Nevertheless, it affords the best access for osteochondritis of the superolateral portion of the dome of the talus, synovial chondromatosis of the ankle laterally and also forms the basis of the Crawford Adams (1948) – or RAF – fusion of the ankle.

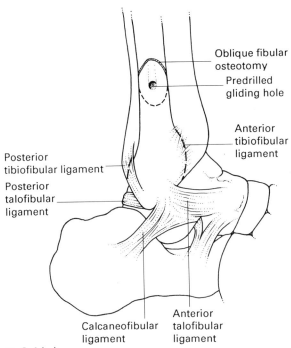

Oblique fibular osteotomy
Predrilled gliding hole
Anterior tibiofibular ligament
Posterior tibiofibular ligament
Posterior talofibular ligament
Calcaneofibular ligament
Anterior talofibular ligament

5.24(a)

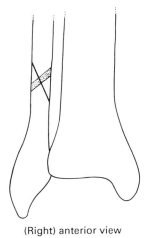

(Right) anterior view

5.24(b)

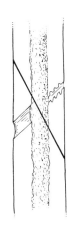

5.24(c)

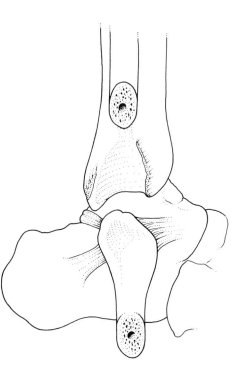

5.24(d)

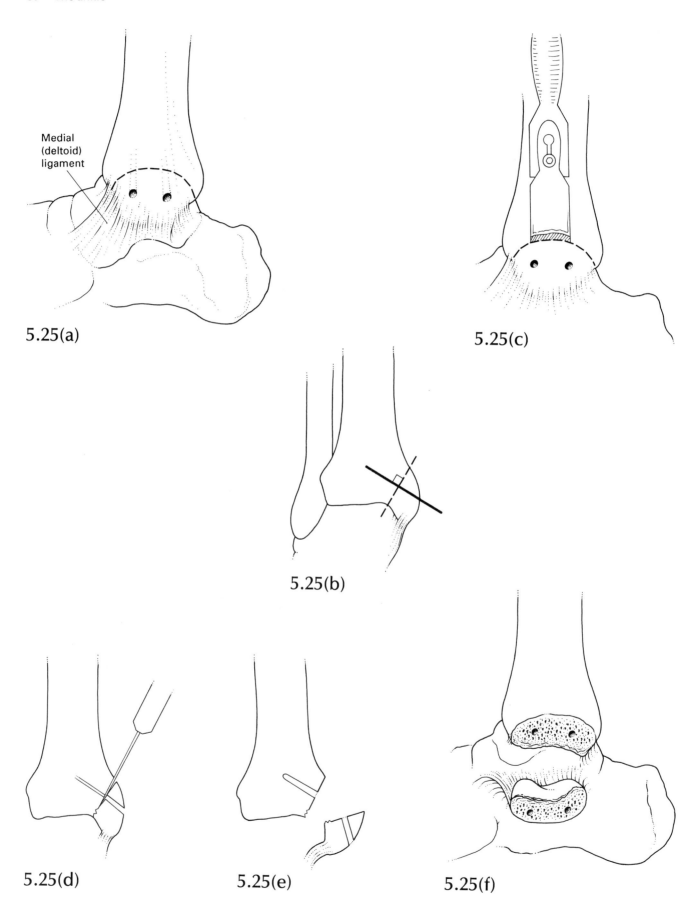

Medial
(deltoid)
ligament

5.25(a)

5.25(b)

5.25(c)

5.25(d)

5.25(e)

5.25(f)

Medial transmalleolar approach (König and Schafer)

Positioning

The patient is positioned supine on the operating table with a foam pad beneath the drapes to support the ankle. A 'sand-bag' beneath the opposite buttock is helpful.

Access

This approach is used to gain entry to the medial part of the ankle joint cavity and the superomedial portion of the dome of the talus.

Incision

This may be the lower portion of either the anteromedial or posteromedial incision. König and Schafer, in fact, described a horizontal incision, slightly convex proximally, at the level of the ankle joint on the medial aspect.

Approach

The principle is to osteotomize the medial malleolus and turn it downwards, hinging on the deltoid ligament. The whole of the base of the medial malleolus is exposed and posteriorly a lever is carefully passed between the bone and the soft tissue structures behind the malleolus. This will serve to protect them, subsequently, from injury during the osteotomy. The near-vertical bony cut is planned to enter the joint at the junction of the horizontal and vertical zones of the tibial articular surface, at the base of the medial malleolus. Two drill holes are made so as to pass through the middle of the proposed bony cut surface, to facilitate later reconstruction, using two cancellous lag screws (Figure 5.25(a),(b)). The bone is then carefully divided with a fine, sharp chisel, along the planned line (Figure 5.25(c)). This requires great care and precision. The subchondral bone adjacent to the site of entry of the osteotomy through the articular cartilage is left uncut and the mobilization of the medial malleolar fragment is completed by osteoclasis to give an irregular,

intra-articular fracture capable of being perfectly restored with the later fixation (Figure 5.25(d)). A minimum of soft tissue mobilization along the edges of the deltoid ligament will then permit downwards tilting of the bony fragment and entry into the ankle joint (Figure 5.25(e),(f)).

Indications

The place for this approach is limited, but it offers a good intra-articular access to the medial side of the ankle for lesions of the superomedial dome of the talus, such as osteochondritis or osteochondral fractures.

References

Adams, J. C. (1948) Arthrodesis of the ankle joint. *J. Bone Joint Surg.*, **30B**, 506

Campbell, W. C. (1949) *Operative Orthopaedics*, 2nd edn, Henry Kimpton, London

Colton, C. L. (1982) *Watson-Jones Fractures and Joint Injuries*, Churchill Livingstone, Edinburgh, p. 1147

Evans, D. L. (1953) Recurrent instability of the ankle – a surgical treatment. *Proc. R. Soc. Med.*, **46**, 343

Gatellier, J. (1931) The juxta-peroneal route in the operative treatment of fracture of the malleolus with posterior marginal fragment. *Surg. Gynecol. Obstet.*, **52**, 67

Gatellier, J. and Chastang (1924) La voie d'acces juxta-retro-péroniere dans le traitement sanglant des fractures malléolaires avec fragment marginal posterieur (technique opératoire). *J. Chir.*, **24**, 513

Glasgow, M., Jackson, A. and Jamieson, A. (1980) Instability of the ankle after injury to the lateral ligament. *J. Bone Joint Surg.*, **62B**, 196

Gordes, W. and Viernstein, Jr, K. (1980) Traitement de l'instabilité tibio-tarsienne par tenodèse à l'aide du court péronier lateral. *Int. Orthop.*, **3**, 293

Konig, F. and Schafer, P. (1929) Osteoplastic surgical exposure of the ankle joint. *Zeit. Chir.*, **215**, 196 (Abstracted in 44th report of *Progress in Orthopaedic Surgery*, p. 17)

Marti, R., Reichen, A., Oberhammer, I. and Raaymakers, E. (1976) Talo-fibular tendon graft for recurrent instability of the ankle joint. In *Injuries of the Ligaments and their Repair*, Chapchal, Theime, Stuttgart, p. 219

Sefton, G. K., George, J., Fitton, J. M. and McMullen, H. (1979) Reconstruction of the anterior talo-fibular ligament for the treatment of the unstable ankle. *J. Bone Joint Surg.*, **61B**, 352

Tillaux (reported by Gosselin) (1872) Rapports recherches; cliniques et experimentales sur les fractures malléolaires. *Bull. Acad. Med. Ser. 2*, **1**, 817

White III, A. A. (1974) A precision posterior ankle fusion. *Clin. Orthop.*, **98**, 239

Chapter 6

The foot

B. Helal

RELEVANT ANATOMY

Incisions on the foot should, where possible, follow natural cleavage lines since they then leave much finer scars.

On the plantar aspect and over the dorsum of the first ray, the cleavage lines are disposed longitudinally. On the lateral aspect of the dorsum they run obliquely from the medial side proximally to the lateral side distally (Figure 6.1).

Peripheral nerves

It is essential to try to avoid section of these since, occasionally, a troublesome neuroma may follow.

The main nerve trunks which supply the foot are detailed in Chapter 5 on the ankle.

SURAL NERVE

This passes into the foot just over 1 cm from the tip of the lateral malleolus and below the peroneal tendons at the base of the fifth metatarsal. It divides into a lateral branch which supplies the dorsolateral surface of the little toe and a medial branch passing obliquely across the dorsolateral surface of the foot, then distally in the fourth interosseous space, where it subdivides to supply the dorsomedial aspect of the little toe and the dorsolateral aspect of the fourth toe.

The sural nerve gives rise to two lateral calcaneal branches, given off just above the lateral malleolus, over the lower quarter of the fibula. The incisions on the lateral aspect should pass in the watershed between this nerve and the superficial peroneal nerve.

SUPERFICIAL PERONEAL NERVE

In the foot this nerve gives off the intermediate dorsal cutaneous nerve which crosses the extensors to the fourth and fifth toes and divides distally in the third cleft to supply the dorsomedial side of the fourth toe and dorsolateral side of the third toe. Its other division is the larger medial dorsal cutaneous nerve. This crosses the extensor retinaculum and runs lateral and parallel to the extensor hallucis longus tendon. It gives off three branches. The medial branch crosses the tendon of extensor hallucis and runs distally on its medial side, anastomosing with the terminal part of the saphenous nerve, to supply the dorsomedial aspect of the great toe. The lateral branch divides distally in the second cleft to supply the dorsomedial aspect of the third toe and the dorsolateral aspect of the second toe. The middle branch divides distally in the first interspace to supply the dorsomedial aspect of the second toe and dorsolateral side of the great toe.

PLANTAR ASPECT OF THE FOOT (Figure 6.2)

The sural nerve supply to the lateral side of the plantar aspect of the heel has been described.

The medial calcaneal branch of the posterior tibial nerve is given off just above the ankle and divides into a

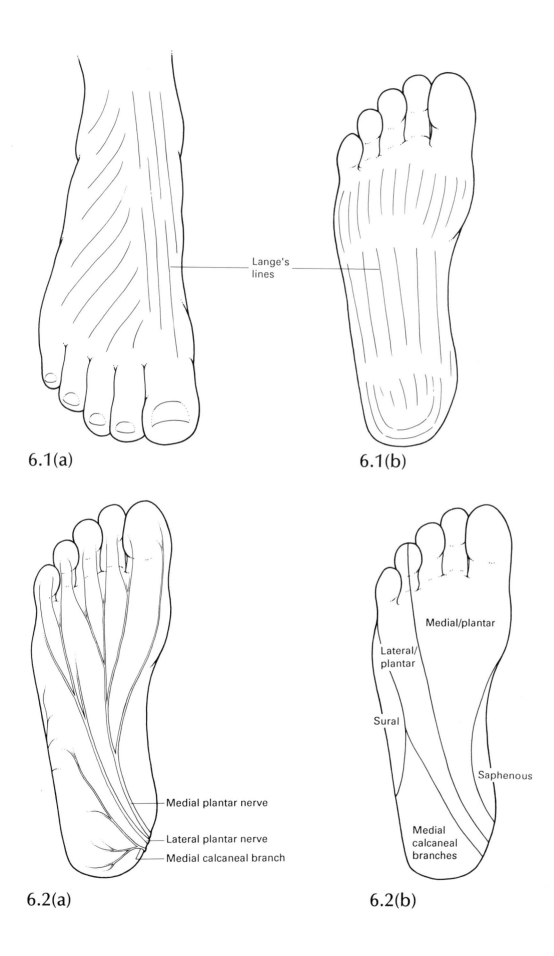

6.1(a)

6.1(b)

Lange's lines

6.2(a)

Medial plantar nerve

Lateral plantar nerve

Medial calcaneal branch

6.2(b)

Medial/plantar

Lateral/plantar

Sural

Saphenous

Medial calcaneal branches

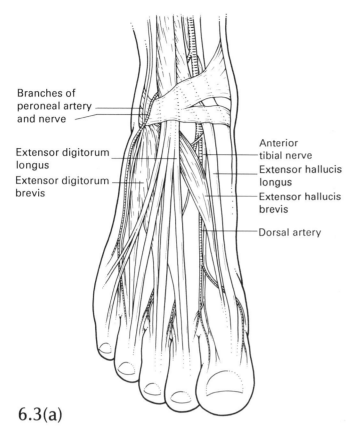

Branches of
peroneal artery
and nerve

Extensor digitorum
longus

Extensor digitorum
brevis

Anterior
tibial nerve

Extensor hallucis
longus

Extensor hallucis
brevis

Dorsal artery

6.3(a)

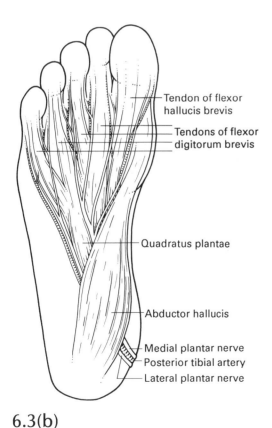

Tendon of flexor
hallucis brevis

Tendons of flexor
digitorum brevis

Quadratus plantae

Abductor hallucis

Medial plantar nerve

Posterior tibial artery

Lateral plantar nerve

6.3(b)

posterior branch, to supply the medial and posterior aspects of the heel, and an anterior branch which supplies the medial side of the plantar aspect. Part of the instep is supplied by the saphenous nerve. The bulk of the sole and plantar aspects of the medial three and a half toes are supplied by the medial plantar nerve; the remainder is supplied by the lateral plantar nerve and a small area of the lateral border by the sural nerve.

The main neurovascular bundle on the dorsum of the foot comprises the anterior tibial vessels and nerve, starting in the centre of the ankle and running forward, between the long extensor of the great toe and the extensor digitorum, to the proximal end of the first intermetatarsal space (Figure 6.3(a)).

The main neurovascular bundles in the sole of the foot run deep to the first layer of muscles, namely the abductors of the great and little toes and the flexor digitorum brevis (Figure 6.3(b)).

SURGICAL APPROACHES

- Anterolateral (Campbell)
- Lateral
- Medial (Henry)
- Plantar incisions
    To the heel
    Medial os calcis
    Plantar sagittal
    Dorsal sagittal
    Dorsal transverse
    Plantar transverse

Anterolateral approach to the ankle and tarsus (Campbell)

Position

The patient is placed supine, with a sandbag beneath the ipsilateral buttock.

Access

The anterolateral approach exposes the anterior aspect of the ankle, the superolateral part of the os calcis, the lateral aspect of the subtalar joint, the sinus tarsi and the calcaneocuboid and talonavicular joints.

Incision

The skin incision begins 3 cm above the lateral malleolus and passes distally, parallel to the anterior border of the fibula, to a point 1 cm below the malleolus, and then curves gently medially across the dorsum of the foot in a line directed towards the base of the great toe. It passes

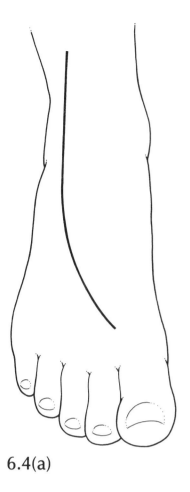

6.4(a)

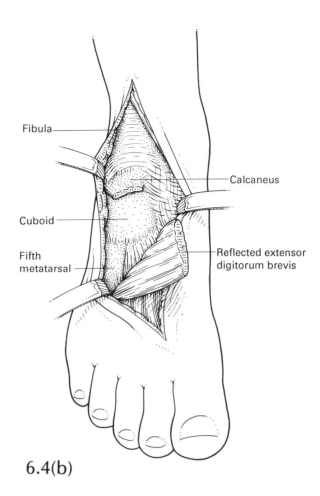

Fibula

Cuboid

Fifth metatarsal

Calcaneus

Reflected extensor digitorum brevis

6.4(b)

dorsal to the peroneal tendons. It lies between the lateral (sural) and medial (superficial peroneal) dorsal cutaneous nerves (Figure 6.4(a)).

Approach

The incision is deepened, dividing the deep fascia and the extensor retinaculum passing just lateral to peroneus tertius and extensor digitorum brevis, which is partially reflected from its origin. The whole of the medial flap thus created is freed from the underlying bones and joint capsules. This interval is developed distally beneath the extensor tendons, which can be elevated and retracted medially. Posteroinferiorly, the peronei are separated from the underlying fascia and retracted posteriorly. The interval thus created exposes the anterior aspect of the ankle, the superolateral part of the os calcis, the lateral aspect of the subtalar joint and the sinus tarsi, the calcaneocuboid joint and the talonavicular joint (Figure 6.4(b)). This approach is the most versatile of the dorsal approaches and gives the greatest access to the tarsal joints. It closes easily and, being in the line of a vascular watershed, heals well.

Indications

This approach may be used for ankle joint replacement or arthrodesis, repair of the anterior tibiofibular ligament and for tarsal fusions. It is not always necessary to use the full extent of the incision.

Lateral approach

Position

The patient is placed supine, with a large sandbag beneath the ipsilateral buttock.

Access

The lateral approach gives access to the os calcis and peronei and to the lateral ligaments of the ankle, the subtalar joint and the base of the fifth metatarsal.

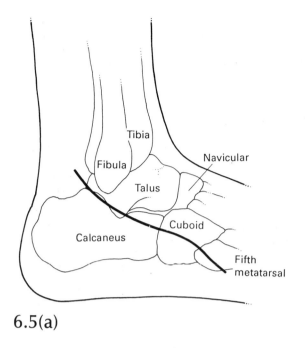

6.5(a)

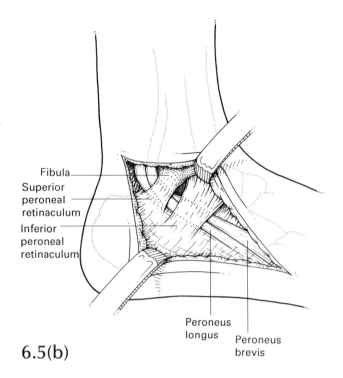

Fibula
Superior peroneal retinaculum
Inferior peroneal retinaculum

Peroneus longus   Peroneus brevis

6.5(b)

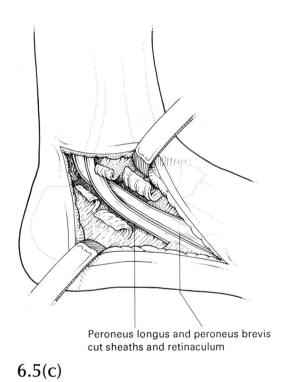

Peroneus longus and peroneus brevis cut sheaths and retinaculum

6.5(c)

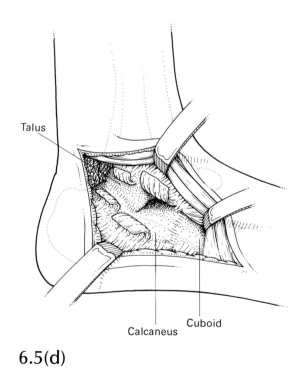

Talus

Calcaneus   Cuboid

6.5(d)

Incision

The skin is incised from a point just anterior to the lateral border of the Achilles tendon and passes obliquely forwards and plantarwards, skirting the apex of the lateral malleolus, then passing across the peroneal tubercle to reach the lower border of the os calcis and the base of the fifth metatarsal (Figure 6.5(a)).

Approach

The incision is deepened by division of the deep fascia (Figure 6.5(b)) and if the peronei need to be retracted, the peroneal sheath is opened (Figure 6.5(c)). Otherwise, the deep incision lies parallel to the peronei, beneath and behind them.

Indications

This incision gives access to the os calcis (Figure 6.5(d)) for elevation and grafting of crush fractures and for osteotomies. It gives access to the peronei and to the lateral ligaments of the ankle.

Medial approach (Henry)

Position

The patient is placed supine with a sandbag beneath the contralateral buttock. With the knee flexed and the hip externally rotated, excellent access is afforded.

Access

The medial approach gives access to the posterior tibial compartment and the medial aspects of both the tarsus and the plantar aponeurosis.

Incision

The skin incision starts 3 cm above the medial malleolus, midway between the tendo Achilles and the postero-medial border of the tibia. It passes down behind the medial malleolus to 0.5 cm beyond its tip and then turns forward towards the base of the first metatarsal (Figure 6.6(a)). Care is taken to avoid damage to the medial calcaneal nerve branches.

Approach

The incision is deepened through the deep fascia and the retinaculum of the posterior tibial compartment and tarsal tunnel with its contained long flexors of the toes and hallux, the tibialis posterior tendon and the posterior tibial neurovascular bundle. Below the medial malleolus, lying on the inner side of the os calcis, is the belly of the abductor hallucis muscle (Figure 6.6(b)) whose tendon passes forward on the belly of the flexor hallucis brevis, distal to the first metatarsal base. The abductor hallucis is hinged plantarwards by partially detaching its origin. The medial plantar nerve and artery are seen on its deep surface. At this point, 2 cm proximal to the navicular tuberosity, the flexor digitorum crosses medial to the flexor hallucis longus tendon. The posterior tibial nerve divides 2 cm below the medial malleolus into lateral and medial plantar nerves. The lateral plantar nerve passes along the lateral border of flexor digitorum brevis. Care to avoid damage to these nerves is important and in this approach it is mandatory to identify and trace them.

The posterior portion of the insertion of tibialis posterior tendon into the navicular tuberosity may be partially lifted anteriorly, ensuring that the elevated tissue remains in continuity with the distal attachments (Figure 6.6(c)).

Indications

This approach gives access to the plantar aspect and medial side of the inner column of bones of the foot, namely the os calcis, navicular, medial cuneiform and first metatarsal, together with the joints between them. It is useful for medial release in club foot and for tarsal tunnel decompression.

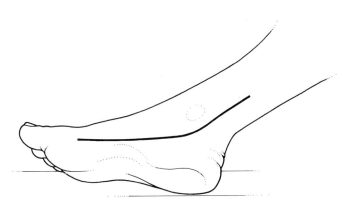

6.6(a)

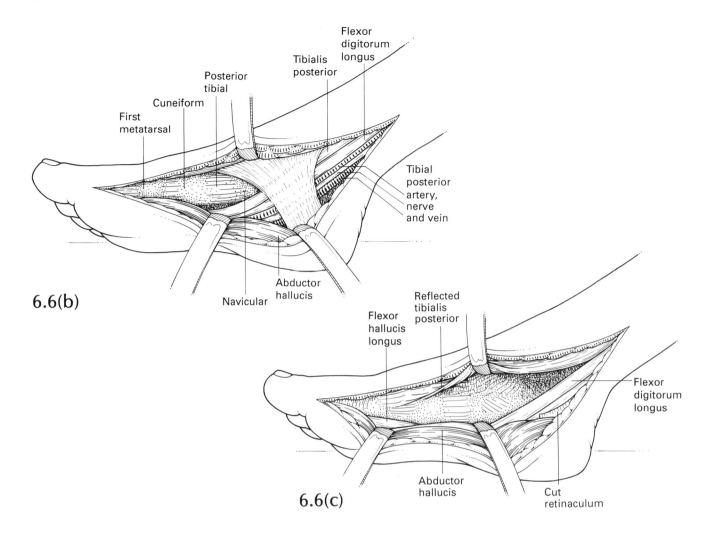

6.6(b)

6.6(c)

Plantar incisions

PLANTAR APPROACH TO THE HEEL

A mid-line incision to the long axis of the foot is made in the heel pad down to the plantar ligament.

Indications

This is rarely indicated other than for exploration of some lesions of the os calcis.

MEDIAL OS CALCIS INCISION

The skin is incised parallel with the inferior bony border of the os calcis.

Indications

Steindler division of the plantar fascia.

PLANTAR SAGITTAL INCISIONS

1. These can be used anywhere on the plantar surface. Two-centimetre incisions, over the appropriate cleft, are used for excision of digital neuromas. The fat is incised and retracted. The deep fascia is then divided to expose the bifurcations of the vessels and nerves to the cleft.
2. A 2-cm incision beneath the first metatarsal head will provide direct access to either sesamoid or to the flexor sheath and the flexor hallucis longus tendon. The flexor sheath is incised and the flexor hallucis retracted away from that sesamoid to be excised.

DORSAL SAGITTAL INCISIONS

Access

Approach to the metatarsal heads and necks from the dorsum.

Incisions

Two-centimetre skin incisions over the first and fifth metatarsals and a single 3-cm incision over the middle metatarsal provide adequate access to the distal thirds of the metatarsals mentioned.

Approach

Dissection proceeds down to the bone using sharp pointed scissors, avoiding section of cutaneous nerves, veins and extensor tendons. Small bone levers are placed round the bone exposed, the soft tissues parted and the bone further exposed proximally and distally by gentle blunt dissection. A sharp periosteal elevator is used to strip the periosteum and interossei from the length of bone to be exposed.

Indications

Osteotomies of the metatarsals (Helal, 1975) and metatarsophalangeal arthroplasties.

DORSAL TRANSVERSE APPROACH

Access

This approach exposes the metatarsal heads and necks and the lesser metatarsophalangeal joints.

Incision

The skin is incised transversely across the line of the metatarsal heads.

Approach

The skin is retracted and the incisions deepened in the sagittal plane on the medial sides of the extensors, down to the dorsal capsules of the joints. These are incised transversely if access to the joint alone is required, or longitudinally if the necks and shafts of the metatarsals also need to be exposed.

Indications

Synovectomy of the metatarsophalangeal joints.*

PLANTAR TRANSVERSE APPROACH

Access

Approach to the metatarsal heads from the plantar aspect.

Incision

A transverse incision is made over the metatarsal necks (Figure 6.7(a)).

Approach

There is usually little subcutaneous fat and the deep fascia and joint capsules are exposed through longitudinal

* Fowler (1959) used this incision for his forefoot arthroplasty, but divided transversely the extensor tendons and dorsal veins. He also excised an ellipse of plantar skin to relocate the fat pad.

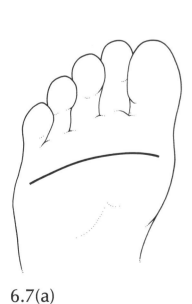

6.7(a)

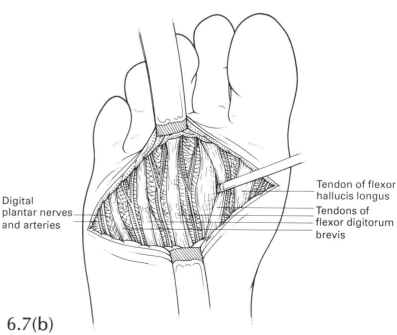

6.7(b)

Digital plantar nerves and arteries

Tendon of flexor hallucis longus

Tendons of flexor digitorum brevis

incisions. The metatarsal head has usually, by virtue of its plantar migration, displaced the vessels and nerves, and sometimes even the flexor apparatus, to one side (Figure 6.7(b)). In any case, care is taken to protect the neurovascular bundles and the flexor apparatus.

Indications

Excision of metatarsal heads and repositioning of a distally migrated metatarsal fat pad, usually in rheumatoid arthritis.

Positions for foot surgery

Supine

Dorsal approaches to the foot are made with a tilt produced by a sandbag or prop to present more of the medial or lateral aspects as required. The sole of the foot can be approached by placing the surgeon at the foot of the table and tilting the table head down.

Prone

Useful for approaches to the sole, the posterior portion of the os calcis and the Achilles tendon insertion.

Plantar grade

This is sometimes necessary to gauge the alignment of the hindfoot in ankle or subtalar surgery. The leg hangs over the table end, as for meniscectomy, but the table is raised high and the foot rests on a trolley with wheel locks. If the trolley is made to move to and fro it is possible to reproduce the ankle movements of walking. By pressure on the knee the foot can be loaded. This position is a useful one for judging the correction of cavus and heel valgus by osteotomies, wedge resections or subtalar prostheses, which otherwise can be extremely difficult.

References

Campbell, W. C. (1956) *Operative Orthopaedics*, 3rd edn, C. V. Mosby, St Louis, p. 195

Fowler, A. W. (1959) A method of forefoot reconstruction. *J. Bone Joint Surg.*, **41B**, 507

Helal, B. (1975) Metatarsal osteotomy for metatarsalgia. *J. Bone Joint Surg.*, **57B**, 187

Henry, A. K. (1959) *Extensile Exposure*, 2nd edn, E. & S. Livingstone, Edinburgh, p. 305

Chapter 7

The spine

J. K. Webb

The format of this chapter differs somewhat from the other chapters in this book, in that it would not be realistic to describe all relevant complex spinal anatomy before the description of each approach. The anatomical structures that it is crucial to recognize during certain approaches will be outlined – their importance and recognition increase the safety of the operation.

- Cervical spine
  Transoral C1–C3
  Mandibular C1–C6
  Extrapharyngeal
  Anterior medial
  Posterior triangle
- Thoracic spine
  Upper thoracic
    Anterior
  Midthoracic
    Thoracotomy
  Lower thoracic
    Thoracoabdominal
- Lumbar spine
  Retroperitoneal
- Posterior approaches
  Cervical
    C1–C2
    C2–C7
  Thoracic
  Lumbar
    Mid-line
    Bilateral paraspinous

CERVICAL SPINE

Anterior approach

The anterior aspect of the upper cervical spine can be approached by two routes – the transoral or the anteromedial. The usual route is via the lateral side of the neck, but it is difficult to visualize C1 and C2 vertebral bodies from this approach, whereas it is relatively easy to reach this area with the transoral access.

TRANSORAL APPROACH

Vertebral artery

The vertebral artery is lateral to the C1 and C2 facet joints.

Position

Under general anaesthesia, with an endotracheal tube, the patient is placed in a supine position with the head in slight hyperextension. A self-retaining mouth retractor, such as a McIver with an accessory blade, is used to hold the mouth open and to retract the endotracheal tube to the side (Figure 7.1). The tongue is sutured away from the surgical route, or packed to one side after insertion of a nasotracheal tube. A tracheostomy is not normally necessary.

If the posterior pharynx is obscured by the soft palate, the uvula can be sutured to the junction of the soft and hard palates. The view of the posterior pharynx may still be difficult, requiring splitting of the uvula in the mid-line and suturing each half to the lateral wall of the oropharynx (Figure 7.2).

Incision

After palpating the posterior pharyngeal wall to identify the anterior tubercle of the atlas, a mid-line 5–6 cm longitudinal incision is made into the pharyngeal raphe, a relatively avascular area.

Approach

There are four layers at this level: posterior phalangeal mucosa, superior constrictor muscle, prevertebral fascia

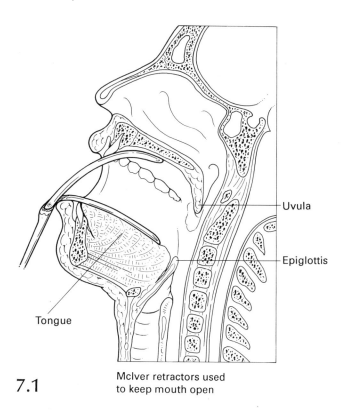

7.1   McIver retractors used to keep mouth open

Uvula

Epiglottis

Tongue

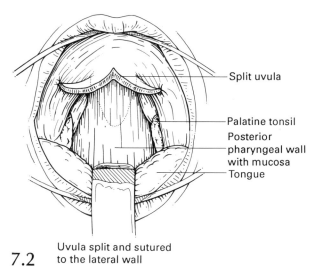

Split uvula

Palatine tonsil

Posterior pharyngeal wall with mucosa

Tongue

7.2   Uvula split and sutured to the lateral wall

and anterior longitudinal ligament. The soft tissues are then stripped laterally as far as the lateral masses of the atlas and axis, using a small swab attached to a Kocher forceps. Stay stitches are placed in the edges of the pharyngeal tissue. Alternatively, particularly if the use of metal is contemplated, then a flap is dissected that is laterally based (Figure 7.3(b)).

This allows adequate exposure from the base of the skull down to the junction of C2–C3 (Figure 7.3(a)). If the base of the skull cannot clearly be seen, the soft palate can be split anteriorly and part of the hard palate removed.

The major fear of this procedure is infection, mainly due to the inability adequately to sterilize the operation field. A further contributory factor may be inadequate closure of the posterior wall of the pharynx. It is important, prior to splitting the pharyngeal raphe, to have an adequate view of the area to facilitate closure. The soft tissues must be closed in two layers. Vertebral artery damage has been described although this artery is behind the lateral mass of the axis and lies on the upper groove of the posterior arch of the atlas (Figure 7.4). If damage occurs, it is usually during resection of bone or tumour.

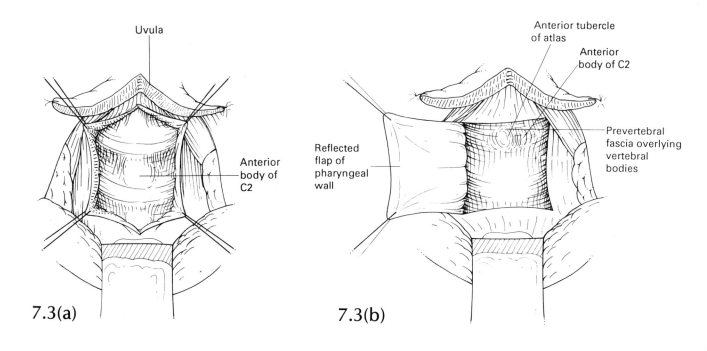

Uvula

Anterior body of C2

7.3(a)

Anterior tubercle of atlas

Anterior body of C2

Reflected flap of pharyngeal wall

Prevertebral fascia overlying vertebral bodies

7.3(b)

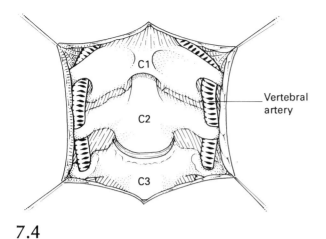

7.4

ANTERIOR APPROACH C1–C6

If anterior exposure between C1 and C6 is required, then the mandibular-tongue-pharyngeal-splitting approach allows an excellent view. This exposure enables one to excise vertebral bodies and tumours. Postoperative infection is kept to a minimum if appropriate antibiotics are prescribed.

Incision

A mid-line, longitudinal skin incision is made (Figure 7.5), and the soft tissues reflected from the mandible.

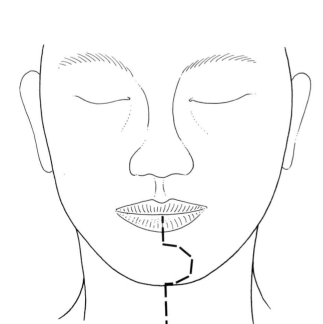

7.5

Approach

A small fragment DCP is contoured and placed onto the centre of the mandible, drilling 2.0 mm holes. The mandible is split in the mid-line (Figure 7.6) and, using electrocautery, the incision continued through the floor of the mouth and mid-line of the tongue as far as the epiglottis (Figure 7.7). Further exposure can be gained by splitting the skin anteriorly as far as the hyoid bone. The

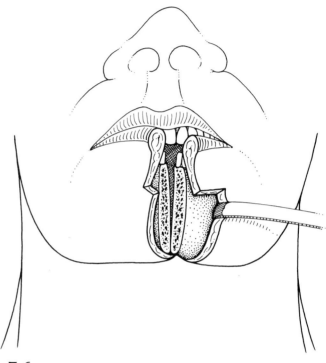

7.6

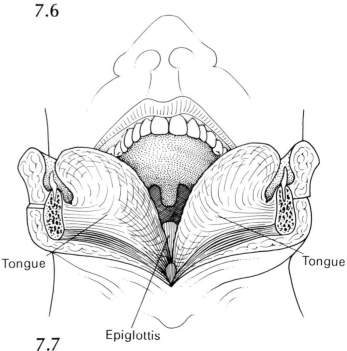

7.7

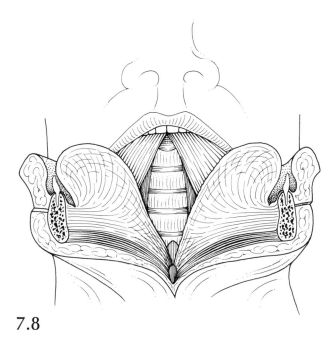

7.8

the internal carotid artery and the ninth, tenth and eleventh nerves. After passing laterally and inferiorly, it emerges superficially between the internal jugular vein and the internal carotid artery below the posterior belly of the digastric muscle, with which it may be confused. It crosses the internal and external carotid arteries and then inclines upwards on the hypoglossus muscle.

Position

Under general anaesthesia, the patient is placed in a supine position with the neck extended and the head rotated to the left.

Incision

An incision is made from the tip of the mastoid process to below the lower edge of the mandible (Figure 7.9). If a more extensive approach to the mid-cervical region is required, then the incision should be curved along the anterior border of the sternomastoid muscle.

soft tissues are reflected laterally and the mucosa of the posterior wall split in the mid-line (Figure 7.8). Closure of the tissues must be performed carefully, with the mucosa closed in two layers.

Approach

The greater auricular nerve should be identified and the platysma incised along the anterior border of the sternomastoid (Figure 7.10). It should be remembered that the sternomastoid muscle is relatively posterior in the upper portion of the spine and the prevertebral strap muscles lie anteriorly.

Identify the carotid sheath by palpation, and note the omohyoid muscle crossing at the level of the cricoid cartilage. It is important to identify the hypoglossal nerve at this level prior to sharp dissection (Figure 7.11). The nerve courses across the front of the external carotid vessels and passes deep to the tendon of the digastric muscle, which can be confused with the hypoglossal

Extrapharyngeal approach to the upper cervical spine

Greater auricular nerve

The largest of the ascending branches of the superficial cervical plexus arises from the second and third cervical nerves. After winding around the back of the sternomastoid muscle and perforating the deep fascia, it ascends with the external jugular vein beneath the platysma (Figure 7.9).

Superior thyroid artery

This artery leaves the external carotid at the level of the hyoid bone, coursing downwards and anteriorly in the carotid triangle along the lateral border of the thyrohyoid. It then passes beneath omohyoid, sternohyoid and sternothyroid, entering the lateral superior aspect of the thyroid.

Hypoglossal nerve

The motor nerve of the tongue must not be damaged. It leaves the occipital bone deep to the internal jugular vein,

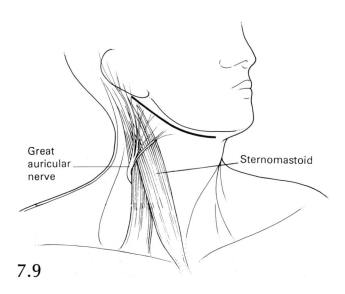

Great
auricular
nerve

Sternomastoid

7.9

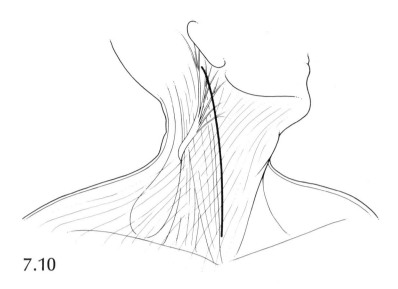

7.10

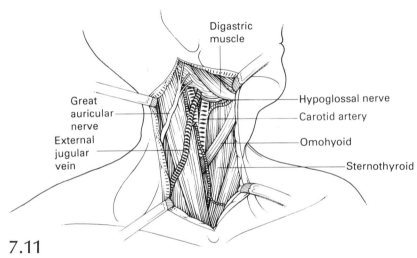

Digastric
muscle

Great
auricular
nerve

External
jugular
vein

Hypoglossal nerve

Carotid artery

Omohyoid

Sternothyroid

7.11

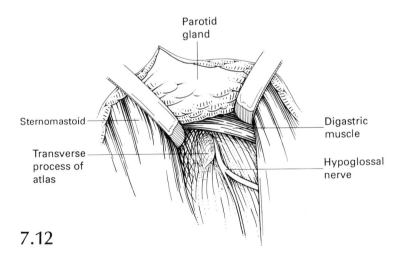

Parotid
gland

Sternomastoid

Transverse
process of
atlas

Digastric
muscle

Hypoglossal
nerve

7.12

nerve. Using blunt dissection, the retropharyngeal space is then entered (Figure 7.12). It is often difficult to enter this space because of the superior thyroid, lingual and facial branches of the external carotid artery which can be divided. If a more extensive exposure is needed, the sternomastoid muscle is detached from the mastoid process, leaving half a centimetre of tissue for later reattachment of the muscle.

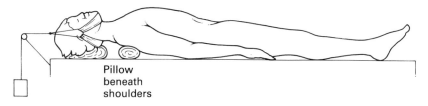

7.13   Halter-traction with the neck in slight traction

Pillow beneath shoulders

Approach to the lower cervical spine – anterior medial

Recurrent laryngeal nerve

This nerve differs on the two sides of the body. On the right side it arises from the vagus nerve in front of the first part of the subclavian artery, coursing posteriorly around the vessel. It ascends alongside the trachea behind the common carotid artery, and is closely related to the inferior pole of the thyroid and the inferior thyroid artery. On the left side, it arises from the vagus coursing below the arch of the aorta, and then ascending to the trachea. The nerve on each side ascends close to the groove between the trachea and the oesophagus.

Carotid artery

The artery passes obliquely upwards from behind the sternoclavicular joint to the upper border of the thyroid cartilage where it divides into the internal and external carotid arteries. The common carotid artery is enclosed in the carotid sheath with the internal jugular vein and the vagus nerve. The superior ramus of the ansa cervicalis is embedded in the anterior sheath.

Superior laryngeal artery

The superior laryngeal artery, frequently a separate branch of the external carotid artery, accompanies the internal laryngeal nerve and passes deep to the thyrohyoid piercing the thyrohyoid membrane.

Superior thyroid artery

This artery arises from the front of the external carotid artery, just below the level of the cornu of the hyoid bone, and divides into terminal branches at the apex of the lobe of the thyroid.

Superior laryngeal nerve

This branch of the vagus nerve descends on the side wall of the pharynx deep to the internal carotid artery. At the level of the hyoid bone, it divides into the internal laryngeal nerve which pierces the thyrohyoid membrane, and a smaller external laryngeal branch which follows the superior thyroid vessels to the side of the larynx.

Thoracic duct

This lymphatic vessel reaches the superior mediastinum from behind the oesophagus. Lying anterior to the intercostal branches of the aorta, it arches across the dome of the left pleura to enter the 'venous angle' of the left internal jugular and subclaviculan veins. It is at risk in approaches from the left below C6.

There is much debate as to whether the approach should be made from the right or left side. The right side is recommended to avoid the thoracic duct, although others would advocate the left side to avoid exposing and damaging the recurrent laryngeal nerve, particularly if the lower cervical spine needs to be exposed.

Position

Place the patient supine with the head rotated 20–30 degrees away from the side to be approached. A head halter applying 10 kg of traction is useful in maintaining slight extension. A small roll is also placed beneath the shoulders (Figure 7.13), and the head stabilized using a 'bean-bag' from which the air has been evacuated.

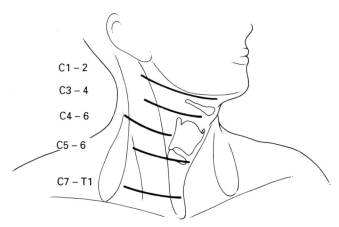

7.14   Level of skin incisions for appropriate levels of the cervical spine

C1 – 2
C3 – 4
C4 – 6
C5 – 6
C7 – T1

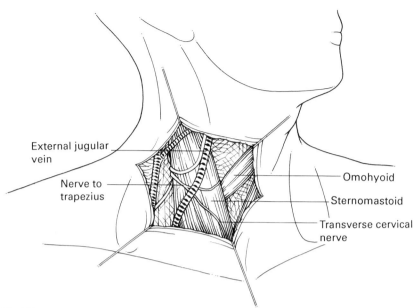

7.15   Medial edge of the sternomastoid identified

Incision

The approach to the cervical vertebrae between the third and the seventh cervical levels presents no serious problem. A transverse, collar incision gives a satisfactory cosmetic scar, but if a more extensive approach is required, an oblique incision along the anterior border of the sternomastoid is recommended. The level of incision will be dictated by the precise vertebral level to be approached (Figure 7.14).

Approach

Continue the incision through the underlying platysma, identify and if necessary ligate the external jugular vein.

The fascia over the anterior edge of the sternomastoid muscle is divided longitudinally. Identifying the anterior border of the sternomastoid is the key to the approach (Figure 7.15).

Soft tissue dissection identifies a space anterior to the muscle edge, and the carotid sheath is then palpated with index finger (Figure 7.16). The oesophagus lies posterior to the trachea and in the superior portion of the neck the larynx is in front of the oesophagus. By gentle blunt soft tissue dissection, the interval is developed between the strap muscles medially and the carotid sheath laterally. The anterior aspects of the vertebral bodies are identified, covered with the prevertebral fascia (Figure 7.17). Incise and retract the fascia longitudinally in the mid-line of the neck. If bleeding from the vertebral bodies is encountered it can be arrested with absorbable bone wax. During exposure of the prevertebral fascia, the inferior thyroid

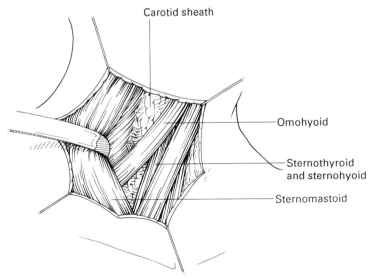

7.16   Carotid sheath identified

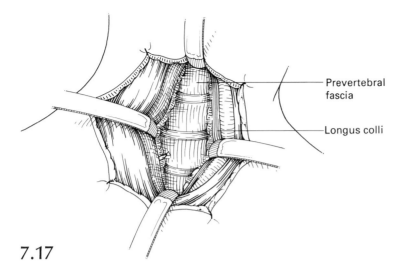

Prevertebral fascia

Longus colli

7.17

vessels should be identified and divided between ligatures. The appropriate cervical level must be identified radiologically at this stage.

The recorded complications particular to this approach are damage to the recurrent laryngeal nerve and perforation to the oesophagus. Provided soft tissue dissection of the prevertebral fascia is performed using swabs, and no sharp dissection is undertaken until the route is clearly identified, then inadvertent injury should not occur.

Posterior triangle approach

Phrenic nerve

The nerve is formed at the upper end of the lateral border of the scalenus anterior, running vertically downwards across the muscle, behind the prevertebral fascia. It descends to the root of the neck behind the sternomastoid.

Brachial plexus

This plexus lies in the posterior triangle of the neck between the clavicle and the lower part of the posterior border of the sternomastoid. It emerges between the scalenus anterior and medius.

Common carotid artery

The artery ascends from behind the sternoclavicular joint to the level of the thyroid cartilage.

Internal jugular vein

At the root of the neck the internal jugular vein lies close to the common carotid artery, slightly laterally, although on the left side it usually overlaps it.

Scalenus anterior

This muscle arises from the anterior tubercles of the transverse processes of the third, fourth, fifth and sixth cervical vertebrae, and, descending almost vertically, is inserted into the inner border of the first rib.

Position

With the patient supine, the neck is extended and rotated away from the side of approach. The head and neck are stabilized using a vacuum 'bean-bag'. The right side is recommended to avoid the thoracic duct (Figure 7.18).

Incision

An incision through skin and platysma is made from the mid-line to the anterior border of the trapezius, 1 cm above the clavicle (Figure 7.18).

Approach

After ligating the external jugular vein, the fascia over the sternomastoid is divided in its lateral half. The posterior triangle fat should be identified, and the carotid sheath palpated (Figure 7.19). Divide the lateral portion of the sternomastoid, after clearing the posterior structures behind the muscle, in particular the internal jugular vein. Retract the carotid sheath and internal jugular vein forward and identify the prevertebral fascia. The scalenus anterior is seen beneath the fascia, with the phrenic nerve crossing its surface from lateral to medial. Carefully dissect this nerve free from the fascia, and retract it medially (Figure 7.20).

One must take care that the sympathetic chain, which lies on the prevertebral fascia, is not damaged. Anterior to the muscle lies the second part of the vertebral artery. Stay medial to approach the spine and remain superficial to the sympathetic plexus and longus colli.

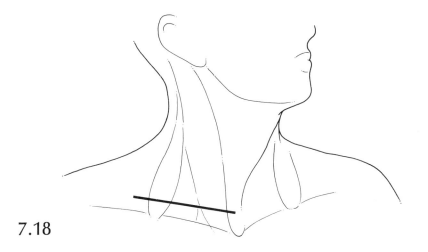

7.18

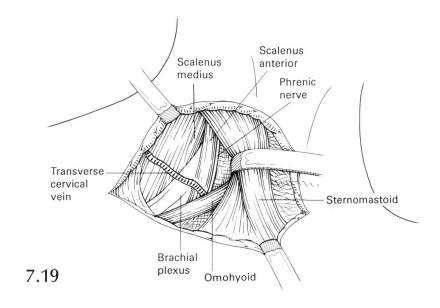

Scalenus
medius

Scalenus
anterior

Phrenic
nerve

Transverse
cervical
vein

Sternomastoid

Brachial
plexus

Omohyoid

7.19

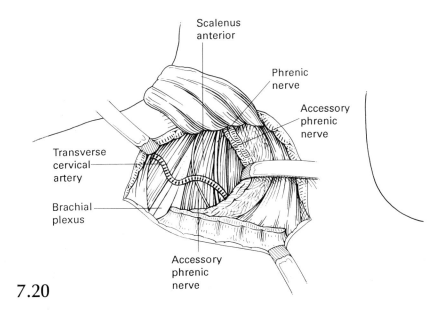

Scalenus
anterior

Phrenic
nerve

Accessory
phrenic
nerve

Transverse
cervical
artery

Brachial
plexus

Accessory
phrenic
nerve

7.20

If a more extensive exposure of the lower vertebra is required, especially the upper thoracic spine, then the scalenus anterior can be divided. Identify the medial and lateral borders of this muscle, lift the muscle from the underlying fascia ensuring the brachial plexus is not injured. Beneath the fascia in the inferior portion of the wound is the apex of the lung. Incising the fascia from the transverse processes of the vertebra allows increased exposure.

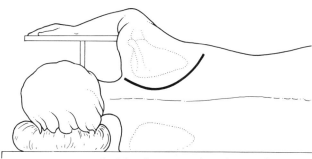

Incision for approach to the anterior aspect of the upper thoracic spine

7.21

THORACIC SPINE

Anterior approach to the upper thoracic spine

Position

The patient is placed in the lateral position, with the uppermost arm supported on an arm-rest in front of the chest and at shoulder level. A right-sided approach is used for preference, as the straight course of the brachiocephalic artery into the base of the neck, compared with the curved course of the left subclavian artery, reduces the likelihood of injury during reflection of the pleura and superior mediastinal structures.

If the pathological lesion lies predominantly on the left side of the spine, a left-sided approach is used.

Incision

The incision begins below the inferior angle of the scapula and curves upwards and medially to finish opposite the spinous process of C7 (Figure 7.21).

At the lower end of the incision, a small portion of latissimus dorsi is divided, including those fibres that insert into the inferior angle of the scapula. Trapezius is divided in line with the skin incision, as medially as possible, in order to minimize the amount of the muscle that will be denervated (Figure 7.22).

Approach

Retract trapezius laterally to expose the rhomboid and levator scapulae muscles as they insert into the medial border of the scapula (Figure 7.23). These muscles are divided and retracted medially, leaving a small portion of each muscle attached to the scapula to facilitate later reattachment.

The scapula can now be retracted laterally exposing the upper chest wall (Figure 7.24). Expose and remove subperiosteally the posterior 7–10 cm of the second, third, fourth and fifth ribs, leaving behind only the head and neck. If only the vertebral body of T2 or T3 is involved, the first rib can usually be left intact, but if exposure of T1 is necessary, the first rib can also be divided with removal of a 2–3 cm segment.

An L-shaped incision is made in the pleura, the lower limb of which is made in the bed of the fifth rib and the vertical limb at the level of the medial cut ends of the ribs. Divide the intercostal muscles, and ligate the segmental neurovascular bundles. Reflect the pleuromuscular flap to enter the pleural cavity. Retraction, or deflation, of the upper lobe of the lung reveals the upper thoracic spine (Figure 7.25).

A combination of blunt and sharp dissection will allow reflection of the pleura and superior mediastinal structures to complete the exposure of the vertebral bodies. Great care must be taken when dissecting around the neck of the first rib to avoid damage to the anterior root of T1 as it crosses to reach the brachial plexus.

Closure

Close each layer, in layers, placing two underwater-seal drains (apical and basal) in the pleural cavity.

The arm is rested in a sling for 2 weeks and the shoulder is then gradually mobilized.

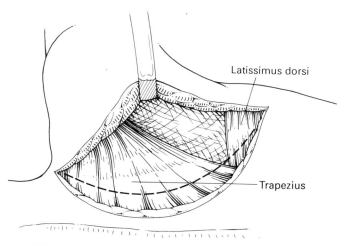

Latissimus dorsi

Trapezius

7.22

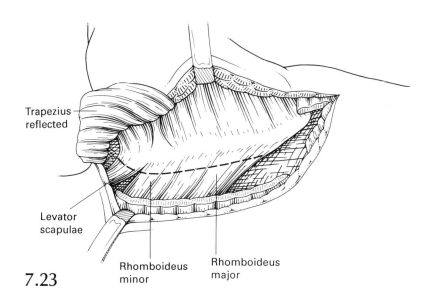

Trapezius reflected

Levator scapulae

Rhomboideus minor

Rhomboideus major

7.23

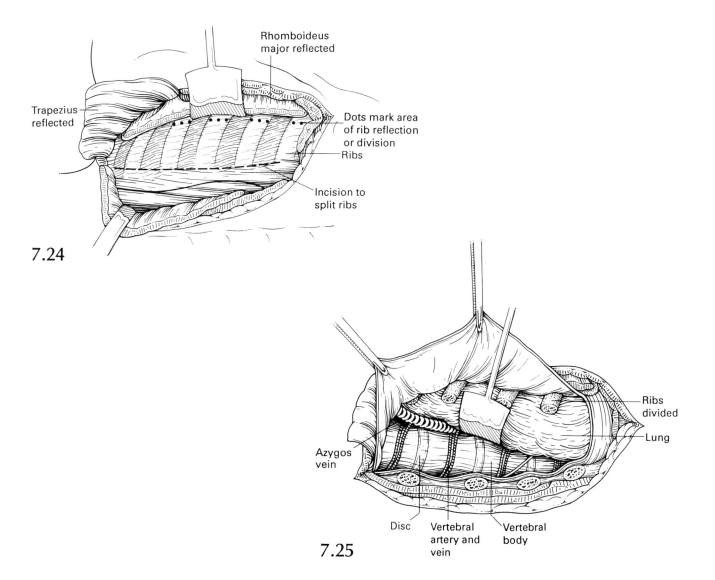

Rhomboideus major reflected

Trapezius reflected

Dots mark area of rib reflection or division

Ribs

Incision to split ribs

7.24

Ribs divided

Lung

Azygos vein

Disc

Vertebral artery and vein

Vertebral body

7.25

Thoracotomy

Intercostal arteries

There are nine intercostal arteries derived from the aorta, supplying the lower nine intercostal spaces, the first two spaces being supplied by the superior intercostal artery. The right posterior intercostal arteries cross the bodies of the vertebra behind the oesophagus, thoracic duct and azygos vein, and are covered by the right lung and pleura. The left arteries run backwards on the vertebrae behind the left lung and pleura. Each artery crosses its intercostal space obliquely towards the angle of the upper rib, coursing forward in the costal groove between the nerve below and vein above. The dorsal branch of the posterior intercostal artery passes posteriorly through a space bounded by the vertebral body medially, above and below by the necks of the ribs and laterally by a superior costotransverse ligament. It gives off a spinal branch, which enters the vertebral canal through the intervertebral foramen, and is distributed to the vertebrae, spinal cord and its membranes.

Sympathetic trunk

This passes in front of the intercostal arteries opposite the heads of the ribs.

Position

The patient is placed in a lateral position, depending upon which side needs to be approached. Approaching the left side is easier, as it is simpler to ligate and divide the vessels arising from the aorta than those draining into the inferior vena cava.

Incision

Identify the precise level of approach by drawing a horizontal line at the appropriate vertebra on a chest

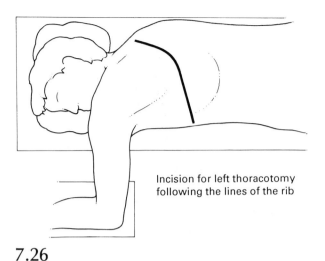

Incision for left thoracotomy following the lines of the rib

7.26

X-ray. The rib transected in the mid-axillary region by this line is the one to be resected, usually two ribs above the vertebral level to which the approach is planned. When the chest is opened, the desired vertebral body is in the centre of the field.

An incision is made from the mid-line posteriorly to the costal cartilage anteriorly (Figure 7.26), dividing the underlying muscles in the same line. It is possible to identify the rib to be approached by either counting from the twelfth or the first ribs, although, with upper thoracic approaches, it is sometimes difficult to identify the first rib. If in doubt, an X-ray should be taken.

Approach

It may well be necessary posteriorly to divide latissimus dorsi, trapezius and rhomboideus major. The periosteum of the rib is split longitudinally, elevated from the superior and inferior portions of the rib, and then carefully lifted from the undersurface of the rib, avoiding damage to the

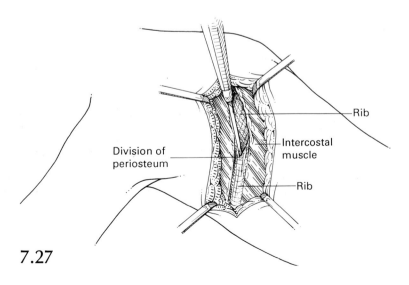

Division of periosteum

Rib

Intercostal muscle

Rib

7.27

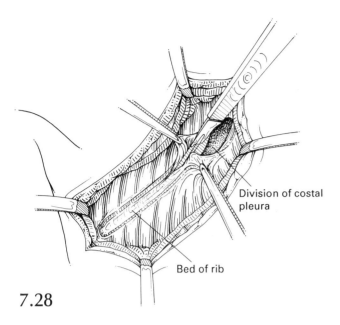

Division of costal
pleura

Bed of rib

7.28

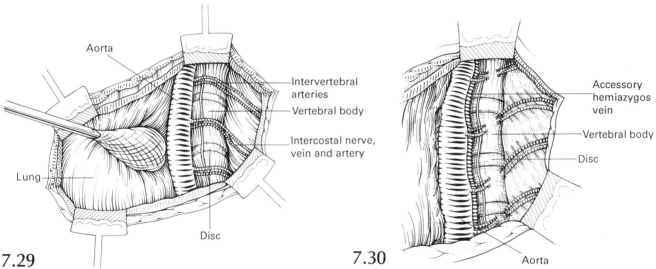

Aorta

Intervertebral
arteries

Vertebral body

Intercostal nerve,
vein and artery

Lung

Disc

7.29

Accessory
hemiazygos
vein

Vertebral body

Disc

Aorta

7.30

intercostal vessels. Resect the rib as far anteriorly and posteriorly as possible (Figure 7.27).

While the lung is deflated, cut the parietal pleura and split this layer gently in line with the rib (Figure 7.28), ensuring that the lung is not adherent to the underlying surface. Retract the lung with a moist gauze swab, and spread the ribs. The vertebral bodies can now be seen, covered with the parietal layer of the pleura, together with the segmental vessels from the aorta and their accompanying veins (Figure 7.29). Gently lift the pleura and split it longitudinally, taking care not to damage the segmental

vessels, which are gently isolated, ligated and divided (Figure 7.30). If the vessels are small, diathermy may be used. The aorta can be pushed gently to the opposite side of the mediastinum and the whole of the spine is then exposed. It is difficult to avoid some damage to the sympathetic plexus. Avoid damaging the dorsal branch of the posterior intercostal artery by not removing the neck of the rib. Do not use diathermy near to the intervertebral foramen to prevent damage to the spinal artery.

The closure of the wound is performed in layers with at least one intercostal pleural drain.

Thoracoabdominal approach, tenth rib

Diaphragm

The diaphragm arises from the xiphoid process, the costal cartilages and adjacent portions of the lower six ribs, the medial and lateral lumbosacral arches and from the two lumbar crura. It is important to recognize the crura; the right, which arises from the anterior bodies and discs of the upper three vertebra, the left from the upper two. Denervation does not occur if the diaphragm is detached around the periphery, as it is supplied centrally by the phrenic nerve.

Genitofemoral nerve

The genitofemoral nerve arises from the first and second lumbar nerves to pass obliquely downwards and forwards through the psoas major. It emerges into the retroperitoneal space near the medial border of psoas opposite the third and fourth lumbar vertebra, before descending on the muscle to the inguinal ligament.

Ureter

The ureter lies behind the peritoneum on the medial border of the psoas major, which intervenes between it and the tips of the transverse processes. It crosses in front of the genitofemoral nerve.

Psoas major

The psoas major arises from the anterior surfaces and tips of all the transverse processes of all the lumbar vertebrae. It proceeds downwards along the brim of the pelvis behind the inguinal ligament to be attached to the lesser trochanter of the femur.

Thoracic duct

Commencing in the cisterna chyli at the T12 level between the aorta and azygous vein, it continues upwards to the right of the aorta between the crura of the diaphragm, to lie to the right of the oesophagus.

Position

The patient is placed in the lateral position. If the pathology allows a choice of approach, the left side is recommended, particularly as the spleen is more easily retracted than the liver.

Incision

An oblique incision is made along the line of the tenth rib, from its posterior aspect to the costal cartilage, and then curving anteriorly to the umbilicus (Figure 7.31).

Approach

Strip the periosteum of the rib along its longitudinal axis. The rib is lifted with a Kocher forceps, and the periosteum stripped from its deep aspect, using a curved periosteal elevator.

Divide the rib as far anteriorly as possible, but do not dissect out the head and neck posteriorly (Figure 7.32). With great care the soft tissue dissection is then carried forward over the costal cartilage towards the mid-line anteriorly. Gentle dissection is used to split the muscles anterior to the costal cartilage. A finger is slipped beneath the cartilage and the peritoneum pushed away from the deep surface of the rib (Figure 7.33). The cartilage is then split in its longitudinal axis and will act as a useful marker when closing the wound (Figure 7.34).

Using a gauze swab, a gap is developed between the peritoneum and the diaphragm. The peritoneum is then swept both from the posterior abdominal wall backwards to the mid-line and from the diaphragm towards the spine. Divide the diaphragm close to the rib, to the mid-line posteriorly, leaving a 2 cm edge for subsequent resuturing (Figure 7.35). The exposure is enlarged by sweeping the peritoneum from the abdominal wall and off the posterior spinal muscles, particularly the psoas, the ureter being carried forwards with the peritoneum. It is sometimes

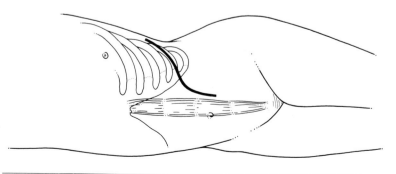

7.31   Incision for the thoracic lumbar approach

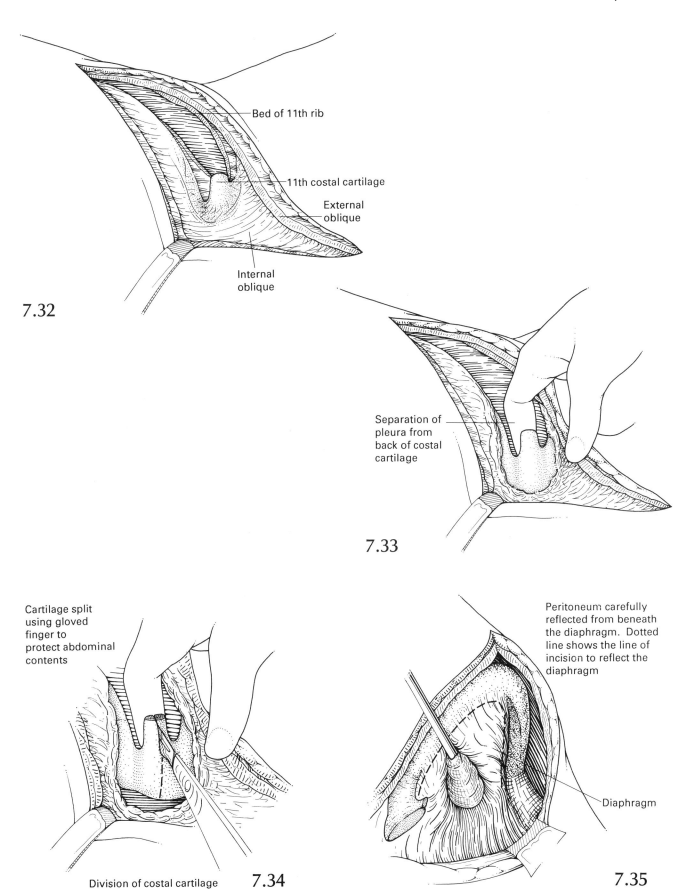

Bed of 11th rib

11th costal cartilage

External
oblique

Internal
oblique

7.32

Separation of
pleura from
back of costal
cartilage

7.33

Cartilage split
using gloved
finger to
protect abdominal
contents

Division of costal cartilage   7.34

Peritoneum carefully
reflected from beneath
the diaphragm. Dotted
line shows the line of
incision to reflect the
diaphragm

Diaphragm

7.35

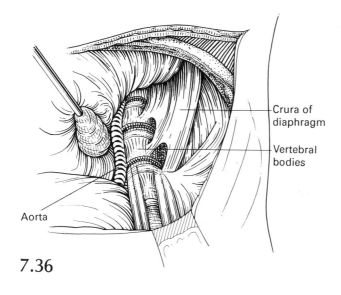

Crura of
diaphragm

Vertebral
bodies

Aorta

7.36

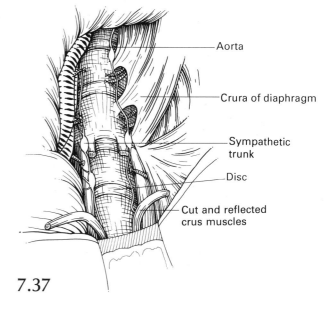

Aorta

Crura of diaphragm

Sympathetic
trunk

Disc

Cut and reflected
crus muscles

7.37

difficult to identify the precise area to be entered underneath the diaphragm, and a useful guide is that the fat in this area is of a loose, 'frothy' consistency, so that as the space is entered, the peritoneum falls away from the muscles very easily. Sharp dissection is not necessary during this procedure and, in fact, would be dangerous as vital structures could be cut. The spine is identified and, in the thoracic region, the parietal pleura lifted and divided longitudinally and the segmental vessels ligated.

Beneath the diaphragm, the diaphragmatic extension (the crus) is divided and lifted from the vertebral bodies (Figure 7.36). If the whole of the lumbar spine needs to be exposed, then the right diaphragmatic crus also is divided, as this extends the exposure to the second lumbar vertebra. An attempt is made to preserve the sympathetic trunk (Figure 7.37).

LUMBAR SPINE

Anterior retroperitoneal approach

Superior hypogastric plexus

The superior hypogastric plexus is situated in front of the bifurcation of the abdominal aorta, the left common iliac vein, the median sacral vessels, the body of the last lumbar vertebra and the promontary of the sacrum. Often referred to as the presacral nerve, it is usually more than one nerve and lies in the extraperitoneal connective tissue. It usually lies to the left of the median line but occasionally lies to the right. If difficulty is encountered in identifying the nerve then infiltration of the area with normal saline will make the plexus easier to identify.

Iliolumbar vein

The iliolumbar vein drains into the common iliac vein and must be identified if the common iliac vein is to be mobilized medially. It courses behind the psoas muscle.

Position

The patient is placed in the lateral position.

Incision

An oblique incision is made between the twelfth rib and the iliac crest from the mid-line anteriorly to a point halfway between the mid-line posteriorly and the mid-axillary region. Depending on the lumbar vertebra to be approached, the incision should either be to the

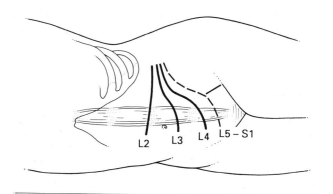

L2   L3   L4   L5 – S1

Appropriate incisions for lumbar vertebrae

7.38

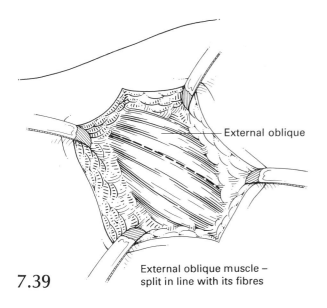

7.39   External oblique

External oblique muscle –
split in line with its fibres

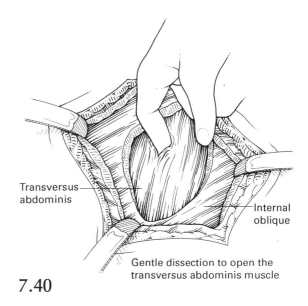

7.40

Transversus
abdominis

Internal
oblique

Gentle dissection to open the
transversus abdominis muscle

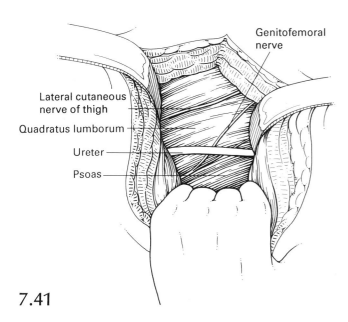

7.41

Genitofemoral
nerve

Lateral cutaneous
nerve of thigh

Quadratus lumborum

Ureter

Psoas

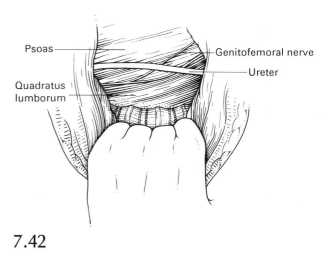

7.42

Psoas

Genitofemoral nerve

Ureter

Quadratus
lumborum

umbilicus or to the junction of the middle and distal thirds of a line between the umbilicus and symphysis (Figure 7.38).

Approach

The muscles are then identified and the external oblique split in the line of its fibres (Figure 7.39). The internal oblique muscle is split in the line of the incision to the edge of the rectus sheath. Open the transversus abdominis muscle by blunt dissection posteriorly so that the retroperitoneal fat becomes visible (Figure 7.40). The peritoneum is stripped from the posterior abdominal wall as far as the mid-line and then the transversus muscle can safely be split. The retroperitoneal fat is loose and the

peritoneum can be stripped from the posterior abdominal wall with ease. It is important to note and protect the genitofemoral nerve and also, as the peritoneum is retracted from the posterior abdominal wall, the ureter (Figure 7.41). Quadratus lumborum and psoas major muscles are easily identified, while medially the vertebral bodies can be felt (Figure 7.42). Identify and ligate the segmental vessels so that the main vessels can be swept away from the mid-line. If the fourth lumbar vertebra needs exposing, it may be difficult to retract the vessels away from the mid-line, and care must be taken to avoid tearing the iliolumbar vein.

If there is the slightest difficulty mobilizing the inferior vena cava and the common iliac vein, the iliolumbar vein should be identified and ligated because, if it is torn accidentally, the resultant bleeding is exceedingly difficult to control (Figure 7.43).

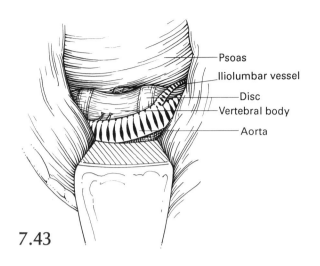

Psoas

Iliolumbar vessel

Disc

Vertebral body

Aorta

7.43

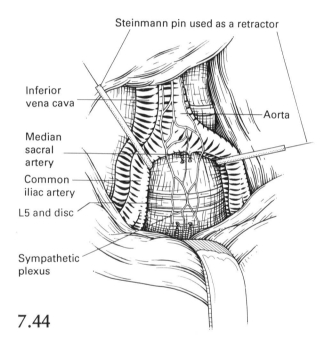

Steinmann pin used as a retractor

Inferior
vena cava

Aorta

Median
sacral
artery

Common
iliac artery

L5 and disc

Sympathetic
plexus

7.44

The mid-lumbar spine is easily visualized. Approach the lumbosacral level between the bifurcation of the great vessels, by sweeping the soft tissues to the right. Blunt dissection should be performed and no neurovascular structure, particularly the presacral nerve, should be divided (Figure 7.44). This is especially important in the male. To aid retraction, two Steinmann pins can be placed in lateral portions of the fifth lumbar vertebral body, to keep the bifurcation apart, allowing ready access to the L5/S1 disc. When inserting the Steinmann pins care should be taken not to damage the vessels, and, in particular, when the Steinmann pin is removed, it is important to ensure that the point does not damage the vessels as it leaves the bone. Bleeding may be encountered from the pin track, and this can be stopped by packing the hole with bone wax.

POSTERIOR APPROACHES

Cervical spine: C1–C2

Vertebral artery

The vertebral artery in this area leaves the foramen transversarium of the atlas to lie on the groove on the upper surface of the posterior arch of the atlas and enters the vertebral canal by passing below the lower arched border of the posterior atlanto-occipital membrane. The dorsal ramus of the first cervical nerve lies between the artery and the posterior arch of the atlas.

Greater occipital nerve

The greater occipital nerve is the large medial branch of the dorsal ramus of the second cervical nerve. It emerges from beneath the inferior oblique muscle travelling upwards to pierce the semispinalis muscle and the trapezius near their attachments to the occipital bone. It communicates with the lesser occipital nerve to supply the back of the skull as far forwards as the vertex.

Position

The patient is carefully prepared and positioned for this procedure, especially if there is spinal instability. Intubation may be facilitated by the fibreoptic endoscope, as the neck must not be flexed if instability exists. 'Log-roll' the patient into the prone position, using a neurosurgical head fixation device attached to the table, ensuring that no pressure occurs on either orbit (Figure 7.45). Skull traction may be required if the neck is unstable. The proposed surgical area is shaved to allow adequate skin preparation. Drapes are sewn into position from the external occipital protruberance to the C4/C5 spinous processes.

Incision

A mid-line incision is made through the skin and the subcutaneous fascia (Figure 7.46).

Approach

The deep dissection should stay in the mid-line raphe to avoid bleeding. Identify the large, bifid spinous process of C2 where the short external rotators to the occiput are attached (Figure 7.47).

Insert a Cobb elevator to face the tip of the spinous process, and sweep down to the base of the spinous process. Reverse the elevator and sweep laterally towards the facet joints. As dissection is carried cephalad, to within half a centimetre of the external occipital protruberance,

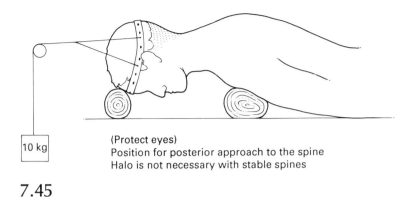

(Protect eyes)
Position for posterior approach to the spine
Halo is not necessary with stable spines

10 kg

7.45

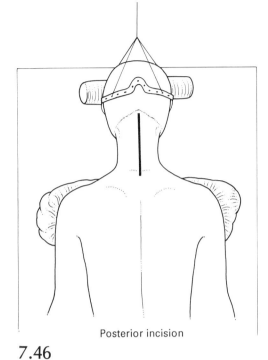

Posterior incision

7.46

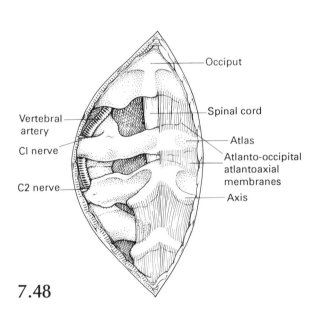

Rectus capitis posterior major

Inferior oblique

Semispinalis cervicalis

Axis of spine

7.47

Occiput

Vertebral artery

Cl nerve

C2 nerve

Spinal cord

Atlas

Atlanto-occipital atlantoaxial membranes

Axis

7.48

the posterior tubercle of C1 is identified. Continue dissecting the lamina of C2 and the occiput laterally.

A sharp, small Cobb elevator is used to clear the ring of the arch of C1 which is slowly stripped laterally (Figure 7.48). *Do not* dissect laterally more than 1.5 cm as beyond this distance is the groove in the lamina for the vertebral artery. The exposure of the occiput, posterior arch of C1 and lamina and spinous process of C2 is now complete. Take care not to damage the greater occipital nerve.

Cervical spine: C2–C7

Incision

A mid-line incision should extend two spinous processes above and two processes below the level to be approached (Figure 7.49).

Approach

Similar preparation is undertaken as for the C1–C2 approach. Cutting diathermy is used to enter the median raphe to minimize bleeding (Figure 7.50).

The spinous processes are identified and exposed and a self-retaining retractor inserted. A Cobb elevator is used to clean the tips of the spinous processes, then reversed, and swept laterally and slightly obliquely caudad to clear the muscle attachments from the lamina. Identify the facet joints (Figure 7.51), pack the area with a swab, and prepare the opposite side in a similar manner. The swabs are then removed and the superficial self-retaining retractors are replaced with deep self-retaining retractors.

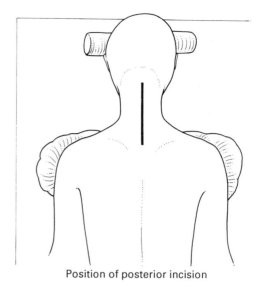

Position of posterior incision

7.49

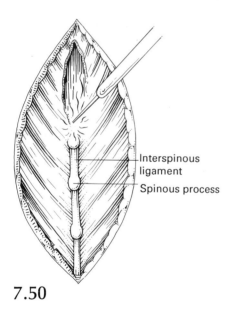

Interspinous ligament

Spinous process

7.50

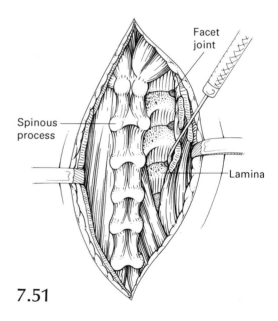

Facet joint

Spinous process

Lamina

7.51

Thoracic spine

Incision

A mid-line posterior incision is made, centred upon the appropriate spinous process. To lessen bleeding, infiltration of the skin and subcutaneous tissue can be performed with sterile 1:500 000 adrenaline solution.

Approach

Cutting diathermy is used to divide the fascia down to the spinous processes, which are identified and cleaned. In the younger patient, the tips of the spinous processes can be split and moved to each side. A Cobb periosteal elevator is used to reflect the muscle subperiosteally from the spinous processes to their bases (Figure 7.52), and then the wound is packed with a swab to secure

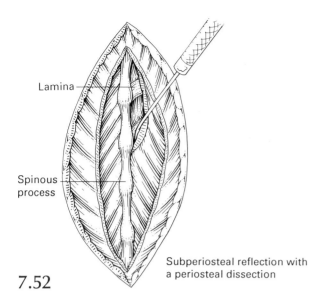

Lamina

Spinous
process

Subperiosteal reflection with
a periosteal dissection

7.52

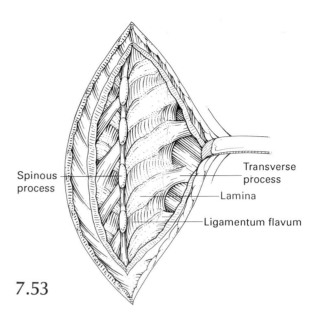

Spinous
process

Transverse
process

Lamina

Ligamentum flavum

7.53

haemostasis. Further dissection is made using the Cobb elevators to detach the muscle origins laterally over the laminae and facet joints to the tips of the transverse processes (Figure 7.53). Pack each side with swabs to secure haemostasis. Diathermy and/or a sharp osteotome may be needed to dissect muscle attachments from the facet area. Dissect each side of the transverse process to its tip, using the Cobb elevator, then divide the muscle around the tip with cutting diathermy. When two adjacent transverse processes have been cleaned, the soft tissue is removed from the facet joint, and the vessels between coagulated.

Lumbar spine

Position

The positioning of the patient is most important. Various

frames are available and whichever apparatus is used, no pressure must be applied to the abdomen (Figure 7.54).

Incision and approach

A similar approach is recommended to that of the thoracic spine but the exposure of the transverse processes is more difficult (Figure 7.55). The laminar area is exposed by using a broad Cobb elevator and sweeping the soft tissues laterally as far as the facet joints (Figure 7.56). A deep self-retaining retractor is inserted lateral to the facet joints. To identify the transverse process, the inferior facet must be identified. A small Cobb elevator is used to clear the tissue from the lamina, the bone is cleaned cranially and the pars interarticularis is identified. Deep to it will be found the base of the transverse process, just inferior and deep to the superior joint facet. With great care the soft

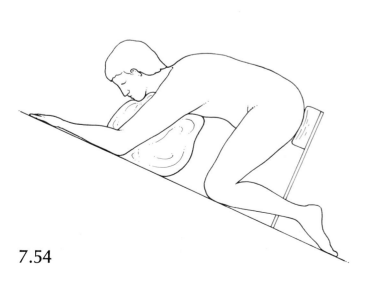

7.54

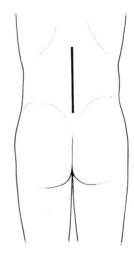

7.55

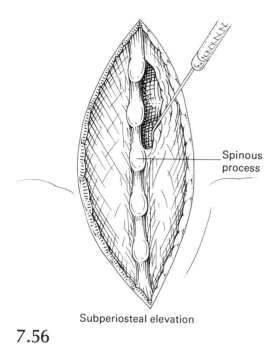

Spinous process

Subperiosteal elevation

7.56

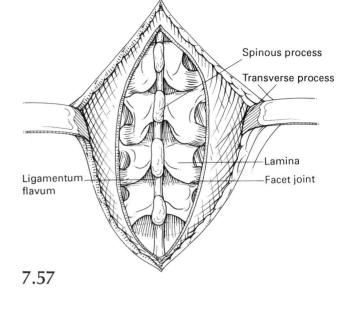

Spinous process

Transverse process

Lamina

Facet joint

Ligamentum flavum

7.57

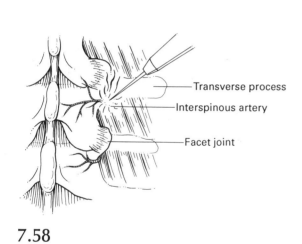

Transverse process

Interspinous artery

Facet joint

7.58

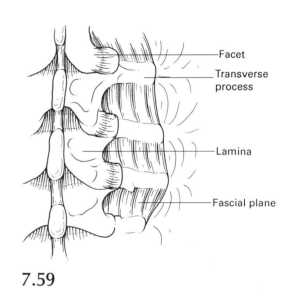

Facet

Transverse process

Lamina

Fascial plane

7.59

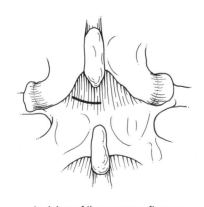

Incision of ligamentum flavum

7.60

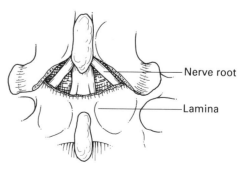

Nerve root

Lamina

7.61

tissue is removed from the transverse process (Figure 7.57), exposing a blood vessel inferior to it, which should be coagulated (Figure 7.58). There is a clear fascial plane between the transverse processes (Figure 7.59).

To enter the spinal canal, cut the ligamentum flavum near the inferior lamina and away from the mid-line (Figure 7.60). Use a fine rongeur to enlarge the opening, exposing the grey/yellow appearance of the extradural fat beneath which lie the nerve roots (Figure 7.61). If necessary, further enlarge the opening either with a curette or by carefully undercutting the adjacent laminar margins with a Kerison rongeur. Identify the pedicle with nerve root exiting caudally around it. The disc is 1 cm cranial to the pedicle.

BILATERAL PARASPINOUS APPROACH

This is a muscle-splitting approach and allows excellent vision of the facet joints and transverse processes, being particularly suitable for an alar transverse fusion.

Position

Position the patient as for the posterior approach to the lumbar spine.

Incision

A curved incision is made on each side three finger breadths lateral to the spinous processes of L4 and S1 (Figure 7.62).

Approach

Expose the lumbar fascia, using a gauze swab to dissect the fat away from the fascia on each side, to aid exposure and closure. The lumbar fascia is cut longitudinally, the transverse processes palpated, and the muscle split down to them (Figure 7.63). Reflect the muscle laterally from the base of the transverse process to the tip and retract with a deep Langenbeck.

The muscle can now be dissected off the facet joints using a Cobb elevator, taking care not to damage the joint above the intended fusion. The gutter between the transverse processes is cleared to the depth of the intertransverse fascia. More medial dissection may be carried out if the ligamentum flavum requires opening.

Further reading

Cloward, R. B. (1958) The anterior approach for removal of ruptured cervical disc. *J. Neurosurg.*, **15**, 602

De Andrade, J. R. and MacNab, I. (1969) Anterior occipital fusion using an extra pharangeal exposure. *J. Bone Joint Surg.*, **51A**, 1621

Fang, H. S. Y. and Ong, G. B. (1962) Direct approaches to the upper cervical spine. *J. Bone Joint Surg.*, **44A**, 1588

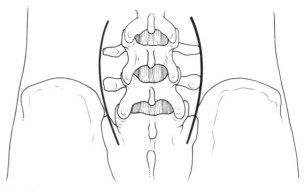

7.62

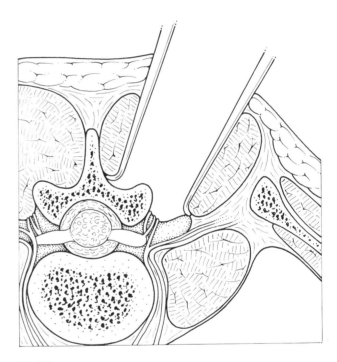

7.63

Henry, A. K. (1957) *Extensile Exposure*, 2nd edn, E. & S. Livingstone, Edinburgh

Hodgson, A. R. and Rau, A. C. M. (1969) Anterior approach to the spinal column. *Recent Adv. Orthop.*, **IX**, 289

Perry, J. (1977) Surgical approaches to the spine. In *The Total Care of Spinal Cord Injuries* (eds D. S. Pierced and V. Nichol), Little, Brown, Boston

Southwick, W. O. and Robinson, R. A. (1957) Surgical approaches to the vertebral bodies in the cervical and lumbar regions. *J. Bone Joint Surg.*, **39A**, 631

Watkins, R. G. (1983) *Surgical Approaches to the Spine*, Springer, New York

Wiltse, L. L., Bateman, J. G., Hutchinson, R. H. and Nelson, W. E. (1963) Paraspinous muscle approach to the lumbar spine. *J. Bone Joint Surg.*, **50A**, 919

Chapter 8

Major neurovascular bundles

R. Birch

SURGICAL APPROACHES

- Supraclavicular approach to posterior triangle of neck
- Display of infraclavicular brachial plexus with great vessels
- Transclavicular approach to cervicothoracic spine and lower roots of brachial plexus
- Emergency exposure of subclavian and axillary artery and vein
- Exposure of circumflex humeral nerve
- Display of brachial sheath
- Display of radial nerve (musculospiral)

Supraclavicular approach to the posterior triangle of the neck

Access

This approach affords access to the spinal nerves and trunks of the brachial plexus, to the accessory and phrenic nerves, to the subclavian artery and to the first thoracic and cervical ribs (if these are present). Medial extension develops the transclavicular approach, and extension in the deltopectoral groove, with or without osteotomy of the clavicle, allows exposure of the retro- and infra-clavicular portions of the brachial plexus, of its terminal nerve trunks, and of the adjacent great vessels.

Position

The patient is placed in a semisedentary position, anaesthetized with a cuffed endotracheal tube. Neuro-

muscular agents are avoided to allow the use of a nerve stimulator. The patient's head is bandaged to a neurosurgical head ring, turned away from the side of approach with the neck in extension. The field of preparation includes the posterior triangle as far as the angle of the jaw and the ear, it extends behind the anterior margin of trapezius and crosses the mid-line of the sternum. The whole of the upper limb is prepared and is left exposed. The chest wall is prepared and exposed down to the inferior margin of the rib cage from the posterior axillary line behind to beyond the mid-line in front. Haemostatic agents may be infiltrated in the line of incision. Bipolar coagulation is used.

Incision (Figure 8.1)

This is a transverse skin crease incision about 2 cm above the clavicle and it extends from the fold of the trapezius behind to the mid-line or beyond in front. Flaps are elevated with the platysma, securing haemostasis and taking care to avoid injury to branches of the supraclavicular nerves (Figure 8.2). The superior flap is elevated to the meeting point of trapezius and sternomastoid and great care is necessary at this point to avoid damage to the accessory nerve. Inferiorly, the flap is raised to expose the insertion of sternomastoid onto the clavicle and the attachments of the deltoid and pectoralis major muscles to the clavicle on its inferior margin (Figure 8.3). Next, the plane between the external jugular vein and the lateral margin of the sternomastoid is developed: this is sometimes difficult when there has been previous surgery or where the posterior triangle is scarred. It is important to find this plane for otherwise the surgeon will easily lose the way! The lateral insertion of sternomastoid may be reflected from the clavicle for a centimetre or two and lifted up as a flap. The omohyoid is the key to the exposure and this muscle is identified and divided across

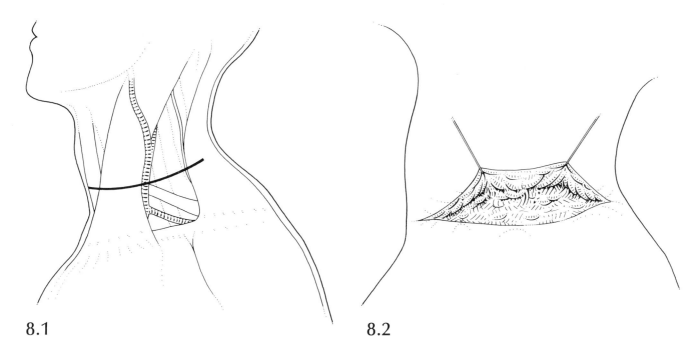

8.1

8.2

its mid-tendinous portion between stay sutures (Figures 8.3, 8.4). The fat pad is now exposed and this is reflected. The transverse cervical vessels are found applied to the deep surface of the fat pad, and they should be identified and ligated. The upper trunk of the brachial plexus is now exposed, gleaming through the investing layer of the prevertebral fascia.

The phrenic nerve will be seen medially, traversing the anterior face of scalenus anterior. This nerve is mobilized from the muscle and held in a light nylon sling. Sharp dissection defines the plane between the upper trunk and

the scalenus medius and then proximally the fifth and sixth cervical nerves are isolated. Distally the suprascapular nerve, passing laterally, is seen and the anterior and posterior divisions of the upper trunk displayed. The seventh cervical nerve will be seen in the interval between scalenus anterior and the upper trunk (Figure 8.5). Troublesome bleeding from veins coursing with the seventh nerve is arrested with bipolar coagulation.

Exposure of the lower trunk of the plexus and of the subclavian artery requires section of scalenus anterior muscle. The position of the artery is easily recognized by

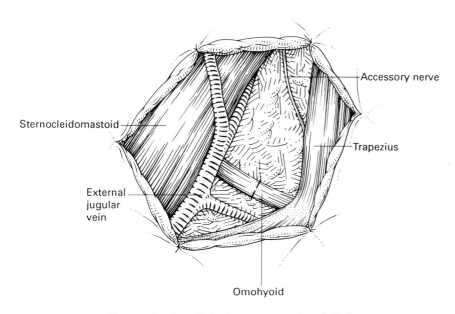

8.3   External jugular vein is shown retracted medially for the sake of clarity; the plane of dissection is between the sternocleidomastoid and external jugular vein

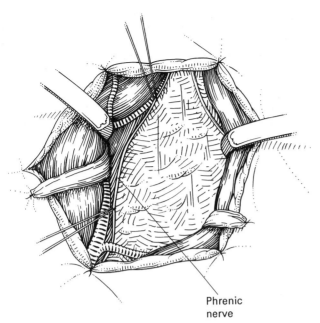

External jugular vein is shown retracted medially for the sake of clarity; the plane of dissection is between the sternocleidomastoid and external jugular vein

8.4

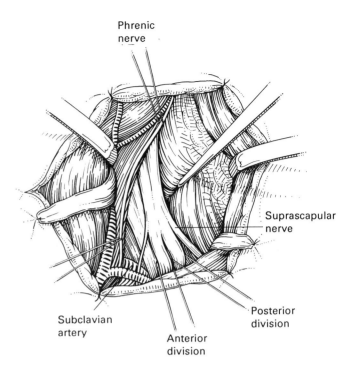

External jugular vein is shown retracted medially for the sake of clarity; the plane of dissection is between the sternocleidomastoid and external jugular vein

8.5

palpation and the plane between it and the muscle in front is gently defined. A malleable retractor passed between the artery and the muscle, with retraction of the phrenic nerve, allows safe division of the muscle. The thyrocervical trunk arising from the subclavian artery is displayed and is ligated and this allows the plane between the lower trunk and the artery to be developed down to the first rib. The suprapleural membrane is seen and is divided and careful subperiosteal dissection of the first rib gives the opportunity to sweep down the pleura, so displaying the eighth cervical and first thoracic spinal nerves and, by medial extension, the thoracic sympathetic chain and stellate ganglion. If the purpose of the operation is to remove a cervical rib or first thoracic rib, then the long thoracic nerve should be displayed and this is easiest seen lateral to the upper trunk within scalenus medius muscle.

Closure

The fat pad is repaired, and omohyoid and sternomastoid muscles reattached. The platysma is closed separately from the skin with interrupted sutures. Two suction drains are recommended, one deep to the sternomastoid and one deep to the platysma.

Complications

A thorough knowledge of the anatomy of the posterior triangle is required for safe work within it. We have seen many iatrogenic injuries of the accessory nerve and of components of the brachial plexus. We have also seen

laceration of the first thoracic nerve in the course of operations for excision of the thoracic rib or of the stellate ganglion. A wound to the external or internal jugular vein risks air embolism; harsh retraction on the trunks of the brachial plexus will be followed by conduction defects. Laceration of the pleura occurs easily if dissection around the first thoracic rib is rough. The subclavian artery must be handled gently and it is customary to secure proximal control using a nylon sling, with an appropriate vascular clamp to hand, before proceeding to full display of the first thoracic or cervical ribs. Section of the terminal branches of the supraclavicular nerves may be followed by painful neuromas.

Display of the infraclavicular brachial plexus with great vessels

A simple infraclavicular approach, through the deltopectoral groove, is useful in a display of the cords, and of the terminal branches, of the brachial plexus. It can be applied in the treatment of benign tumours of those trunk nerves, of isolated ruptures of such nerves as the axillary and the musculocutaneous, and in certain wounds. However, the approach is usually an extension of the supraclavicular method, which is described above.

is considerable variation in the disposition of nerve trunks at this level, particularly for the musculocutaneous and median nerves. The musculocutaneous nerve may pass into coracobrachialis as little as 1 cm distal to the coracoid process, and it is at risk here. Control of bleeding from the axillary artery is sometimes difficult because of the overlying median nerve. Incisions through skin previously irradiated for cancer may not heal, and the supraclavicular and infraclavicular incisions are best separated in such patients.

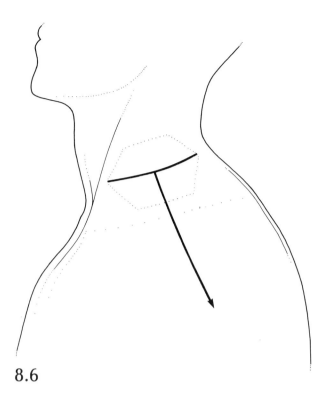

8.6

Incision

The incision for supraclavicular exposure is extended as a 'T' into the deltopectoral groove (Figure 8.6). The cephalic vein is displaced laterally for the exposure of structures medial to the coracoid and the vein is displaced medially if access to the glenohumeral joint is required, as in cases of Erb's palsy. The clavipectoral fascia is incised longitudinally (Figure 8.7). The pectoralis minor tendon is divided about 1 cm from its insertion onto the coracoid after ligation of the thoracoacromial leash (Figure 8.8). The axillary artery and vein, and the three cords of the plexus are now displayed (Figure 8.9). Osteotomy of the clavicle is necessary to secure display of retroclavicular injury to the brachial plexus and to the subclavian vessels and also for extensive tumours. Where retroclavicular injury is recent, then the usual fracture of the clavicle provides the osteotomy. In other cases, a strong nylon tape passed about the clavicle is sufficient to allow access.

Wound closure

Pectoralis minor is reattached and then a few sutures are used to approximate the margins of the deltopectoral groove. If the clavicle is osteotomized or if there is an associated, recent fracture, then this is stabilized with a contoured small fragment compression plate.

Complications

The field is cramped, particularly in muscular patients, and partial release of pectoralis major may be necessary. There

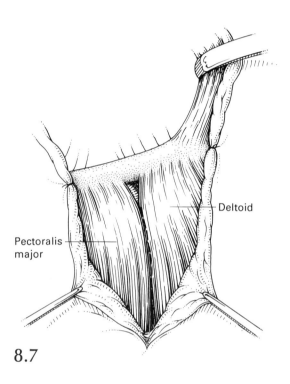

8.7

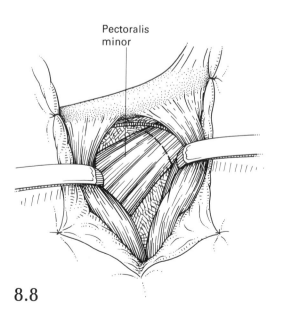

8.8

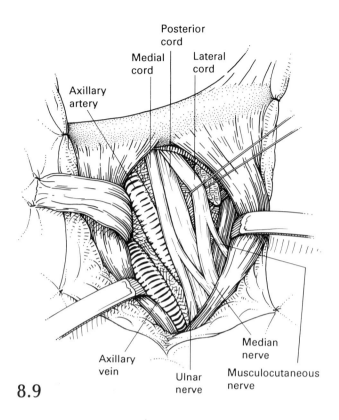

Posterior cord
Medial cord
Lateral cord
Axillary artery
Axillary vein
Ulnar nerve
Median nerve
Musculocutaneous nerve

8.9

Transclavicular approach to the cervicothoracic spine and the lower roots of the brachial plexus

The display of the cervicothoracic junction of the lower roots of the brachial plexus is difficult and approaches such as the lower cervical (Perry, 1977), costotransversectomy (Capener, 1954), sternal split (Cauchoix and Binet, 1957) and the posterior thoracotomy (Turner and Webb, 1987) all have limitations. We favour an approach developed by Bonney (1990), similar to an exposure of the deep vessels attributed to Duval by Fiolle and Delmas (1921). There are similarities too, to a recent description for approach to the upper dorsal spine by Charles and Govender (1989).

In this operation an osseous flap containing the medial half of the clavicle and the upper corner of the manubrium sterni, together with the intervening sternoclavicular joint, is elevated on the sternocleidomastoid muscle and section of the first costochondral junction is necessary. Where possible the approach should be from the left side as on the right side the recurrent laryngeal nerve crosses the field and is vulnerable to injury from traction. The more difficult right-sided approach is illustrated here.

Position

The patient is positioned as for the supraclavicular approach to the posterior triangle. Skin preparation is similar but more extensive including both posterior triangles, the chin and both mandibles, and the anterior chest wall.

Incision

This is T-shaped with the transverse limb in the skin crease 2 cm above the clavicle and the vertical limb in the mid-line extending midway down the sternum (Figure 8.10). Flaps are raised to include platysma extending to the hyoid bone above and sufficient to expose the clavicle on the side of approach below. The skin flaps are sutured into position (Figure 8.11). The supraclavicular nerves are identified and protected wherever possible but medial branches sometimes have to be divided. Care must be taken to avoid damage to the accessory nerve. The investing layer of cervical fascia is incised along both anterior and posterior margins of the sternocleidomastoid muscle which is defined and separated from deeper structures (Figures 8.12, 8.13). Pectoralis major is separated from the clavicle as far as the sternoclavicular joint (Figure 8.14). The superior aspect of the manubrium sterni is defined and the first costal cartilage displayed.

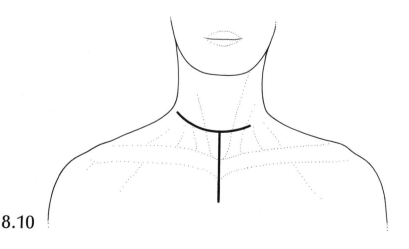

8.10

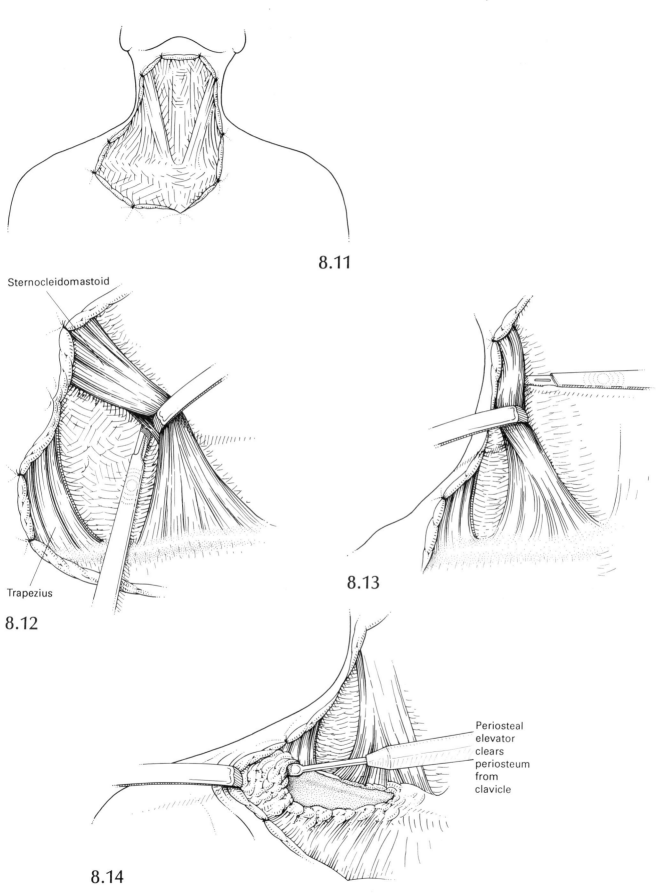

8.11

Sternocleidomastoid

Trapezius

8.12

8.13

Periosteal
elevator
clears
periosteum
from
clavicle

8.14

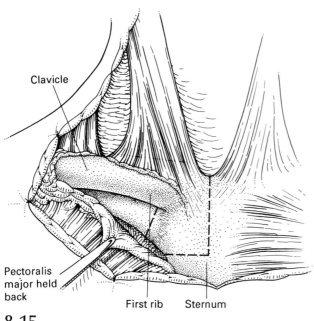

Clavicle

Pectoralis
major held
back

First rib   Sternum

8.15

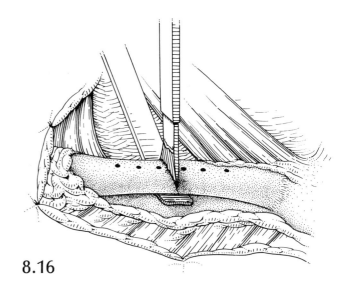

8.16

Malleable rectractors are now passed deep to the sternum and the upper outer quadrant of the manubrium is divided carefully with osteotomes; the first costal cartilage is divided with a scalpel, again after passing a malleable retractor deep to it (Figure 8.15). The mid-point of the clavicle is osteotomized after predrilling screwholes for later application of a previously contoured plate (Figure

8.16). The bone flap is now elevated on the sternocleido-mastoid muscle.

The omohyoid muscle is now defined and divided to display the internal jugular vein and common carotid artery (Figure 8.17). Exposure of the lower roots of the brachial plexus and of the subclavian artery is achieved by division of the scalenus anterior, after retraction of the phrenic nerve (Figures, 8.18, 8.19).

Access to the cervicothoracic junction is by development of the plane medial to the carotid sheath, displacing

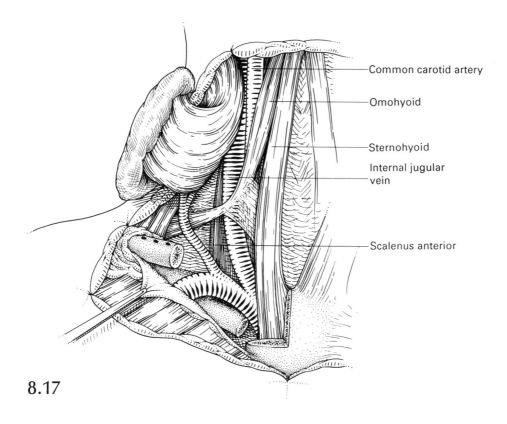

Common carotid artery

Omohyoid

Sternohyoid

Internal jugular
vein

Scalenus anterior

8.17

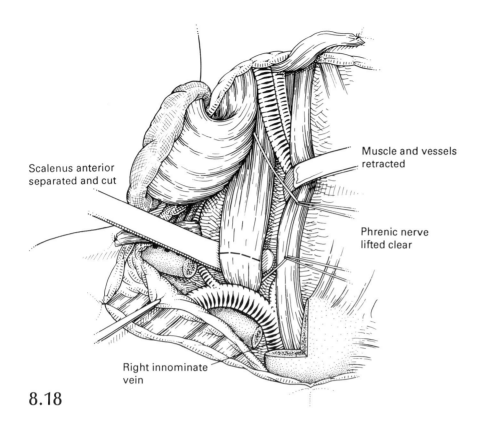

Scalenus anterior
separated and cut

Muscle and vessels
retracted

Phrenic nerve
lifted clear

Right innominate
vein

8.18

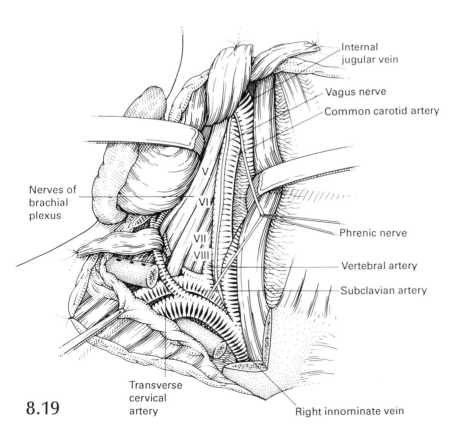

Internal
jugular vein

Vagus nerve

Common carotid artery

Nerves of
brachial
plexus

V

VI

VII

VIII

Phrenic nerve

Vertebral artery

Subclavian artery

Transverse
cervical
artery

Right innominate vein

8.19

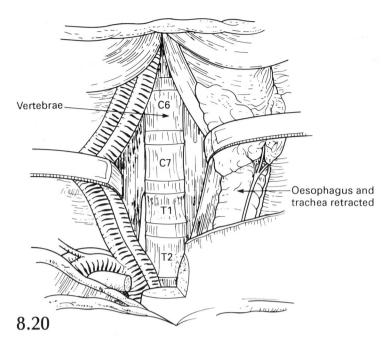

Vertebrae

C6

C7

T1

T2

Oesophagus and
trachea retracted

8.20

the trachea and oesophagus to the opposite side (Figure 8.20). The recurrent laryngeal nerve may be damaged by traction or pressure and is particularly vulnerable on the right side because of its shorter course.

This approach allows an excellent display of the brachial plexus from the spinal column to the formation of the cords, of the subclavian and carotid vessels and of the great vessels at the root of the limb. Anterior access to the dorsal spine down to the disc space between T3 and T4 is achieved and instrumentation down to the body of T3 is possible.

Closure

The flap of manubrium is reattached with wires and the first costal cartilage may be sutured. The clavicle is stabilized by a previously contoured compression plate. Pectoralis major and omohyoid muscles are repaired. Several suction drains are used, both superficial and deep. The platysma is sutured separately from the skin.

Complications

The chief danger from this operation is impairment of ventilation. Planned tracheostomy is used in those patients where there is extensive removal of bone to allow anterior decompression of the spinal cord. In other cases, endotracheal intubation is advised for at least 24 hours after the operation and lateral radiographs are useful in indicating oedema or haematoma deep to the trachea. Laceration of the pleura may occur and a radiograph of the chest to exclude pneumothorax is necessary. The exposure is extensive and close attention to replacement of blood loss and to the risks of air embolism is vital. This operation is a difficult one but the exposure achieved, and the safety gained by display and control of the great

vessels, amply justify its use in certain complex cases of nerve tumour extending into the spinal canal, of tumours arising from the spinal column, or of vascular abnormality.

Note: One patient in 26 of the author's series died from disseminated intravascular coagulopathy and there has been one case of recurrent laryngeal palsy which ultimately recovered. Intercostal drains were necessary in six patients.

Emergency exposure of the subclavian and axillary artery and vein

In cases where these vessels have been injured lateral to scalenus anterior there can be no doubt that the best exposure is that described by Fiolle and Delmas (1921) and discussed by Henry (1973). The elements of this have been discussed already (see p. 122) and include the transverse supraclavicular incision with a T-shaped extension into the deltopectoral groove. The incision is through the skin and platysma only, with exposure of the clavicle. The inferior margin of the pectoralis major muscle is defined, then released from the humerus and reflected medially. Pectoralis minor is released and the clavicle divided with a Gigli saw. This operation allows rapid and safe access to injured nerves and vessels between the inferior margin of pectoralis minor and the lateral margin of scalenus anterior. Release of the lateral part of sternomastoid and of scalenus anterior extends access to the proximary part of the subclavian artery and subclavian vein. This operation is preferred to excision of the clavicle which is time consuming and functionally unacceptable. The common practice of incision along the line of the subclavian–axillary axis through pectoralis major leads to massive scar formation and denervation of the pectoralis muscle. Whilst resection of the medial portion of the clavicle has, on occasion, been performed, we feel that the transclavicular approach is the better operation, but a thorough knowledge of that operation is necessary.

Exposure of the circumflex humeral nerve

Open wounds of the circumflex nerve are uncommon but rupture from traction injury to the brachial plexus, dislocation of the shoulder or fractures of the humeral neck, is more frequent. In such cases, the proximal neuroma is invariably found anteriorly, just below the coracoid, and two incisions are necessary to expose both proximal and distal stumps.

The anterior stump is best displayed through the infraclavicular exposure of the brachial plexus (see p. 123). The posterior incision is made from the proximal insertion of the deltoid muscle to the posterior axillary fold (Figure 8.21). The deltoid is separated from the underlying teres minor, triceps, infraspinatus and teres major muscles. The circumflex nerve is then seen passing through the quadrilateral space together with the circumflex artery and vein (Figure 8.22). This combined anterior and posterior approach is invariably needed when the nerve is to be repaired by graft passed through the quadrilateral space before suture to anterior and posterior stumps.

Closure

The deltoid cowl is replaced and lightly sutured. Subcuticular suture of the skin gives the best cosmetic result.

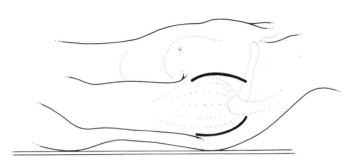

8.21

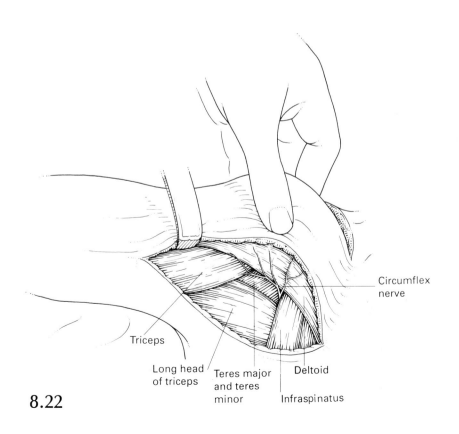

8.22

Circumflex nerve

Triceps

Long head of triceps

Teres major and teres minor

Deltoid

Infraspinatus

Display of the brachial sheath

This exposure is commonly used to gain access to the medial cutaneous nerve of the forearm for grafting. An excellent exposure of the proximal part of the radial nerve is given before the nerve passes round the spiral groove. In severe traction ruptures of the neurovascular axis, the distal stump of the axillary artery and of the main nerve trunks often recoil into the brachial sheath.

Position

The patient is placed supine with the shoulder abducted to 90° and the arm supported on a table.

Incision

This curves into the axilla from just below the pectoralis major muscle and then continues along the medial aspect of the arm over the natural sulcus between the triceps and biceps muscles (Figures 8.23, 8.24). The inferior border of the pectoralis major muscle is carefully defined. This then allows the axillary fat pad to be swept down, exposing the brachial sheath where it emerges from the axilla. The brachial sheath is a well-defined envelope. The first nerve to be seen is the medial cutaneous nerve of the forearm which is adherent to a brachial vein (Figure 8.25). The nerve perforates the sheath in the middle part of the arm.

In the upper part of the wound the ulnar nerve is seen medial to the brachial artery and underneath the brachial vein, but halfway down the arm the nerve pierces the intermuscular septum and runs along the surface of the medial head of the triceps (Figure 8.26). The median nerve crosses over the brachial artery from its lateral to its medial side. The radial nerve crosses the latissimus dorsi tendon at the apex of the incision and one or two motor branches to triceps accompany it. The musculocutaneous nerve lies in a plane between coracobrachialis and biceps muscles and by lifting up the pectoralis major muscle the nerve can be seen passing from the lateral cord into the elbow flexors (Figure 8.27).

This exposure is a logical extension of the infraclavicular exposure described above. Distal extension to display the

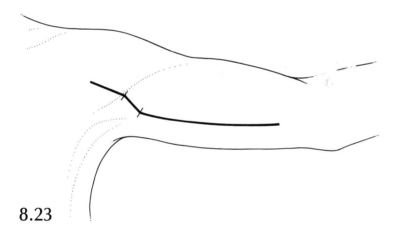

8.23

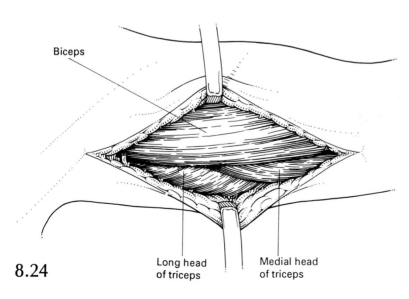

8.24   Biceps

Long head of triceps   Medial head of triceps

ulnar and median nerves is also possible. It is a useful incision for displaying the most proximal part of the radial nerve, where that has been ruptured by fracture of the shaft of the humerus.

Complications

The median and musculocutaneous nerves often follow a variable pattern and the musculocutaneous nerve may pass into the elbow flexor muscles as a separate trunk, even as distal as the mid-arm. The ulnar nerve frequently gives small branches supplying the medial head of the triceps. Injury to the small distal branches of the medial cutaneous nerve of the forearm should be avoided, for these frequently give rise to extremely painful neuromas.

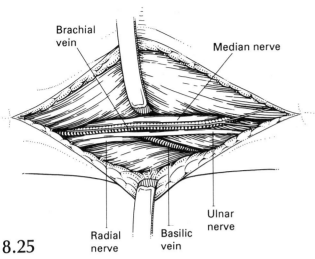

8.25

Brachial vein · Median nerve · Radial nerve · Basilic vein · Ulnar nerve

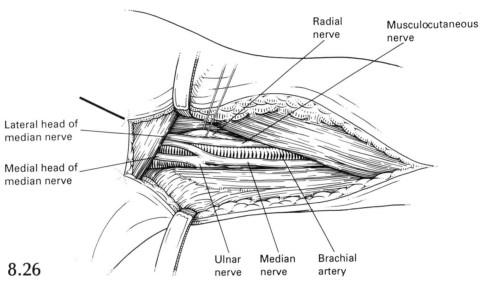

8.26

Radial nerve · Musculocutaneous nerve · Lateral head of median nerve · Medial head of median nerve · Ulnar nerve · Median nerve · Brachial artery

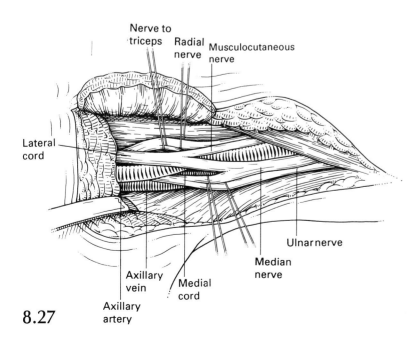

8.27

Nerve to triceps · Radial nerve · Musculocutaneous nerve · Lateral cord · Axillary vein · Medial cord · Ulnar nerve · Median nerve · Axillary artery

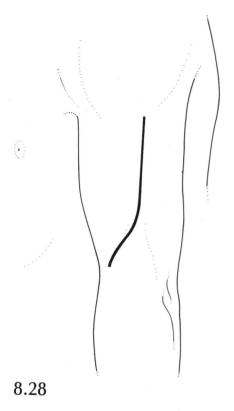

8.28

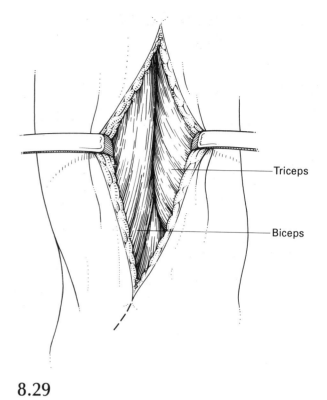

Triceps

Biceps

8.29

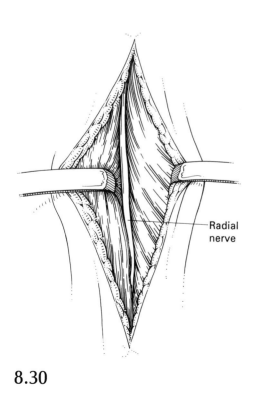

Radial
nerve

8.30

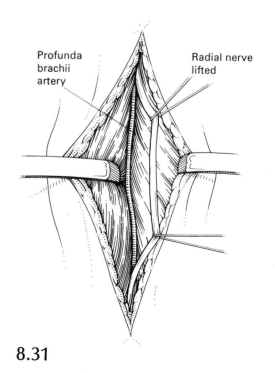

Profunda
brachii
artery

Radial nerve
lifted

8.31

Display of the radial nerve (musculospiral)

The radial nerve is one of the most commonly injured peripheral nerves. It may be damaged in closed fractures of the humerus and it is also, unfortunately, vulnerable during operations to stabilize fractures of the humerus, or during the course of operations to remove plates. The proximal part of the radial nerve is easily displayed through the brachial incision with extension into the axilla previously described (see p. 131). Where the limb is scarred from previous fractures or operation then the safest display for the distal part of the radial nerve is by entering the plane between the brachialis and brachioradialis muscles just above the elbow (Figures 8.28, 8.29). From here the nerve can be traced distally to its bifurcation into posterior interosseous and superficial radial nerves. The nerve trunk can be traced proximally to the level of lesion. Bleeding from the associated vessels may be tedious. Branches to brachioradialis and to extensor carpi radialis longus pass laterally and the safest plane for dissection is between the radial nerve and brachialis muscles (Figures 8.30, 8.31).

References

Bonney, G., Birch, R. and Marshall, R. W. (1990) A surgical approach to the cervico-thoracic spine. *J. Bone Joint Surg.* **72B**, 904–907

Capener, N. (1954) The evolution of lateral rachotomy. *J. Bone Joint Surg.*, **36B**, 173–179

Cauchoix, J. and Binet, J. P. (1957) Anterior surgical approaches to the spine. *Ann. R. Coll. Surg. Engl.*, **35**, 237–243

Charles, R. W. and Govender, S. (1989) Anterior approach to the upper thoracic vertebrae. *J. Bone Joint Surg.*, **71B**, 81–84

Fiolle, J. and Delmas, J. (1921) In *The Surgical Exposure of Deep Seated Blood-vessels* (ed. C. G. Cumston), Heinemann, London, pp. 61–67

Henry, A. K. (1973) *Extensile Exposure*, Churchill Livingstone, Edinburgh, pp. 15–47

Perry, J. (1977) Surgical approaches to the cervical spine. In *The Total Care of Spinal Injuries* (eds E. S. Pierce and V. H. Nickel), Little, Brown, Boston

Turner, P. L. and Webb, J. K. (1987) A surgical approach to the upper thoracic spine. *J. Bone Joint Surg.*, **67B**, 542–544

Further reading

Fang, H. S. Y., Ong, G. B. and Hodgson, A. R. (1964) Anterior spinal fusion. The operative approach. *Clin. Orthop.*, **35**, 16

Louis, R. (1983) *Surgery of the Spine*, Springer, Berlin

MacRae, R. (1987) *Practical Orthopaedic Exposures*, Churchill Livingstone, Edinburgh, pp. 24–50

Van den Brink, K. D. and Edmondson, A. S. (1980) The spine. In *Campbell's Operative Orthopaedics* (eds A. S. Edmonson and A. H. Crenshaw), C. V. Mosby, St Louis

The shoulder

W. A. Wallace

RELEVANT ANATOMY AND PATIENT POSITIONING

Joints at the shoulder

The shoulder region encompasses two true joints – the glenohumeral joint and the acromioclavicular joint. In addition there is one unusual 'joint' – the subacromial joint – which allows the supraspinatus tendon and greater tuberosity to slide under the coracoacromial arch formed by the acromion posteriorly and the coracoacromial ligament anteriorly (Figure 9.1). The function of the glenohumeral joint depends on the muscles around the shoulder functioning well and of these the deltoid is the most important. The deltoid cloaks the shoulder region (Figure 9.2) and must be either retracted, split longitudinally or repositioned to give access to the

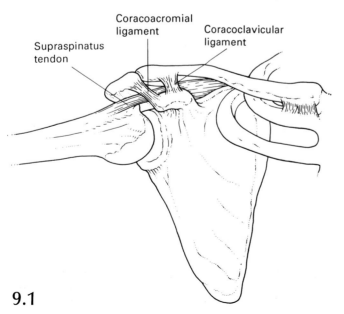

9.1

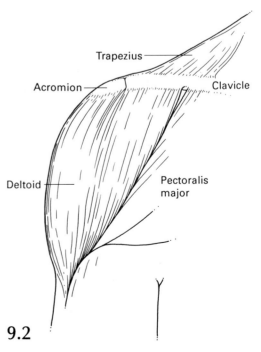

9.2

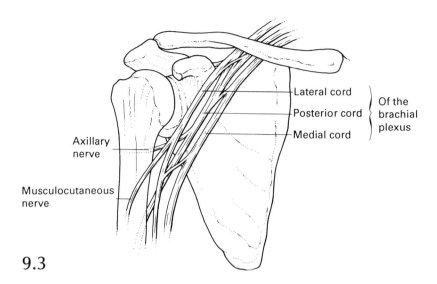

9.3

glenohumeral and subacromial joints. The deltoid should
not be detached from its origins (the lateral third of the
clavicle, the acromion and the lateral spine of the scapula)
unless absolutely necessary for exposure, as repair of the
deltoid origin is difficult and, more importantly, the soft
tissue repair will delay the start of the postoperative
physiotherapy regimen.

Nerves at risk

Three nerves are particularly at risk during operations in
the region of the shoulder:

ANTERIORLY (Figure 9.3)

The musculocutaneous nerve leaves the lateral cord of the
brachial plexus opposite the lower border of the
pectoralis minor muscle. It passes laterally giving one or
two small twigs to the coracobrachialis muscle, pierces
that muscle about 7 cm distal to the tip of the acromion
and runs down laterally in the groove between the biceps
and the brachialis muscles to reach the lateral side of the
arm where it ends as the lateral cutaneous nerve of the
forearm. It may be traumatized due to traction as it passes
through coracobrachialis or it can be caught in sutures
inserted inferior to the glenoid.

INFERIORLY (Figure 9.4)

The axillary nerve which supplies the deltoid and teres
minor muscles is at risk as it passes around the back of the
neck of the humerus. It can be located 5 cm distal to
the tip of the acromion where it passes through the
quadrilateral space and then into the deltoid muscle.
Finally, as the lateral cutaneous nerve of the arm, it

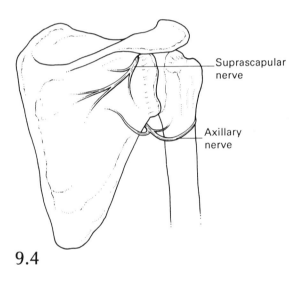

9.4

provides the sensory supply over the lateral aspect of
the upper arm.

POSTERIORLY (Figure 9.4)

The suprascapular nerve may be damaged as it proceeds
around the scapular notch at the lateral end of the spine
of the scapula when passing from the supraspinatus to
the infraspinatus muscles.

Positioning

The shoulder region is very mobile, being attached to
the axial skeleton by only the clavicle and soft tissues.
Positioning of the patient prior to surgery is therefore

very important to steady the area to be exposed and allow easy access. Two standard positions are used for shoulder surgery – the dental chair (sometimes called the astronaut) position for all anterior and superior surgery and the lateral position for posterior surgery.

DENTAL CHAIR POSITION (Figure 9.5)

This ensures the shoulder is well elevated by adjusting the trunk to a 45 degree tilt, thus reducing venous pressure and the risk of bleeding. The shoulder is stabilized by placing a small sand-bag (or 500 ml plastic saline infusion bag) under the medial border of the scapula. This is the ideal position for most shoulder operations and is used by most shoulder surgeons throughout the world.

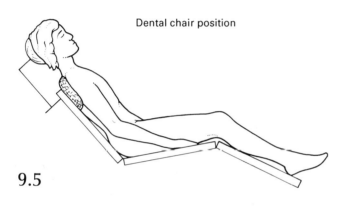

Dental chair position

9.5

LATERAL POSITION (Figure 9.6)

This again ensures elevation of the shoulder region and allows access to both the back and the front of the shoulder. The trunk must be stabilized with a padded vertical post anteriorly against the lower chest cage and posteriorly with a firm pad applied to the middle of the thoracic spine. This position is used both for posterior shoulder surgery and for arthroscopy of the shoulder.

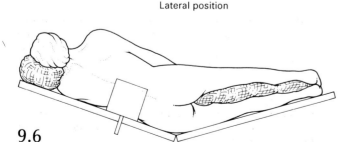

Lateral position

9.6

SURGICAL APPROACHES

- Anterior deltopectoral
- Long anterior deltopectoral (Neer, Watson and Stanton, 1982)
- Anterior extensile (Redfern, Wallace and Beddows, 1989)
- Axillary
- Deltoid-splitting transacromioclavicular joint (Ha'Eri and Wiley, 1981)
- Transacromial (Kessel, 1982)
- Posterior
- Coronal for acromioclavicular joint
- Parasagittal for acromioclavicular joint

Anterior deltopectoral approach

Access

This exposure is the standard method of access to the front of the shoulder for shoulder stabilization operations for recurrent anterior dislocation or for exploration of the glenohumeral joint. The anterior glenoid rim can be exposed, but access to the rest of the glenohumeral joint and the humeral neck is limited.

Incision (Figure 9.7)

A vertical incision 8 cm long is made through skin from the tip of the coracoid down towards the anterior axillary fold. The incision is deepened through fat to the fascia overlying the deltoid and pectoralis major.

Approach (Figure 9.8)

The distal part of the incision crosses the deltopectoral groove and careful dissection will reveal the cephalic vein lying within the groove. The deltoid and pectoralis major are separated with the cephalic vein retracted medially, and side branches are ligated as necessary. If there is difficulty in dissecting the cephalic vein it may be ligated at the proximal and distal ends. Self-retaining retractors are inserted to separate the deltoid and pectoralis major muscles (Figure 9.9). The coracoid is now exposed at the proximal end of the incision and the conjoined tendon of the short head of biceps and the coracobrachialis is identified. A small cruciate incision is made over the tip of the coracoid which is predrilled with a 2.5-mm diameter drill along the length of the distal part. The direction of drilling is determined by palpation of the coracoid. The depth of the hole is then measured, tapped with a 3.5-mm tap and thus prepared for reattachment later with a 4.0-mm small cancellous screw. The soft tissues are divided across the coracoid 1.5 cm from its tip and haemostasis achieved before division of the coracoid is carried out with an

Anterior deltopectoral approach

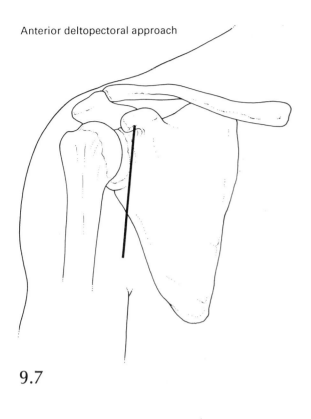

9.7

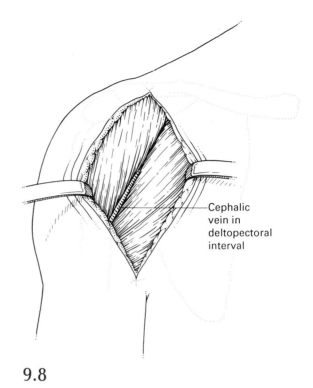

Cephalic
vein in
deltopectoral
interval

9.8

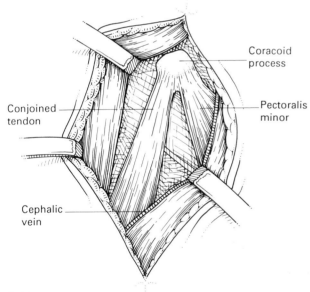

Coracoid
process

Conjoined
tendon

Pectoralis
minor

Cephalic
vein

9.9

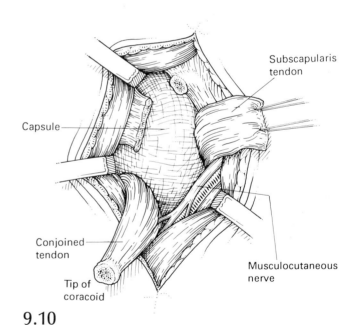

Subscapularis
tendon

Capsule

Conjoined
tendon

Tip of
coracoid

Musculocutaneous
nerve

9.10

osteotome. The divided tip of the coracoid is gently retracted downwards and soft tissue dissected away from the conjoined tendon, taking care to preserve the musculocutaneous nerve at its medial edge, approximately 4–6 cm distal to the coracoid. The coracoid and conjoined tendon should now be gently placed in a subcutaneous pocket just inferior to the distal end of the incision. It is important to avoid unnecessary traction which may result in injury to the musculocutaneous nerve (Figure 9.10). The subscapularis tendon

overlies the front of the humeral head. Its upper border is identified by palpation just inferior to the base of the coracoid and its lower border by a leash of veins running along this border which communicate with the anterior circumflex humeral veins. These veins should be cauterized and the anterior capsule separated from the subscapularis by gentle blunt dissection. Two stay sutures should now be inserted into the subscapularis to control retraction and its tendon divided 2 cm from its lateral attachment. By external rotation of the arm the anterior capsule is brought into view and can be divided vertically to expose the glenohumeral joint and the anterior rim of the glenoid.

Indications

This approach is used for surgical repair of recurrent anterior dislocation of the shoulder. It may also be used for removal of loose bodies, drainage of a septic arthritis and for limited synovectomy. Coracoid osteotomy is optional but makes the exposure of the deeper structures much easier.

Long anterior deltopectoral approach

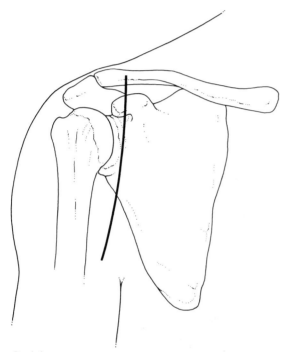

9.11

Long anterior deltopectoral approach (Neer, Watson and Stanton)

Access

This approach provides an exposure of the front of the glenohumeral joint, the upper humeral shaft and the humeral head.

Incision (Figure 9.11)

A 17-cm incision is made from the clavicle down across the tip of the coracoid and continued in a straight line to the anterior border of the insertion of the deltoid.

Approach (Figure 9.12)

The cephalic vain is ligated distally and proximally, high in the deltopectoral groove. The deltoid is retracted laterally and the arm abducted 40–60 degrees. The clavipectoral fascia is incised. The subacromial space is cleared and a broad elevator is placed beneath the acromion as a retractor. At this stage improved exposure will be obtained by either dividing the proximal 1.5 cm of the insertion of pectoralis major as recommended by Cofield (R. H. Cofield, 1983, personal communication), or by releasing the anterior insertion of deltoid as advised by Neer. The shoulder is flexed and externally rotated to facilitate coagulation of the anterior circumflex humeral vessels. Stay sutures are inserted into the

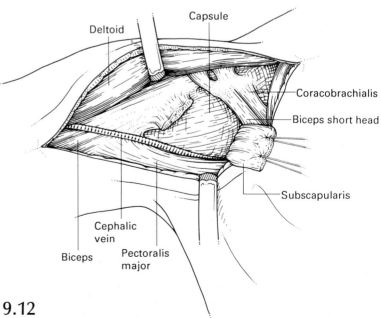

9.12

subscapularis muscle to control retraction and its tendon is divided 2 cm medial to the bicipital groove (Figure 9.12). If the subscapularis appears tight it should be divided in an oblique or 'Z' manner to allow repair with lengthening of the tendon. The joint capsule is then released anteriorly and inferiorly whilst taking care to protect the axillary nerve with a blunt elevator where it passes through the quadrilateral space. The glenohumeral joint may now be dislocated anteriorly by abduction and external rotation, allowing a full exposure of the humeral head and neck.

Indications

This exposure gives moderate access to the head and neck of the humerus which is sufficient for humeral hemi-arthroplasty or total shoulder replacement. It is currently the approach recommended by Neer for total shoulder replacement.

Anterior extensile approach

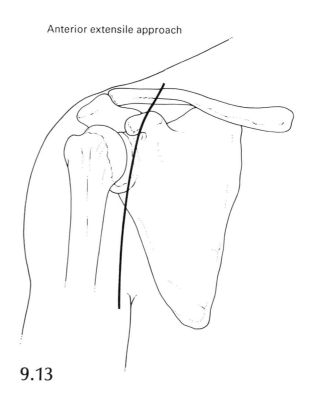

9.13

Anterior extensile approach (Redfern, Wallace and Beddows)

Access

This approach allows a wide exposure of the whole of the front of the shoulder region, providing access to the glenohumeral joint, the whole of the humeral head, the subacromial region and the humeral neck distally as far as the insertion of deltoid. It is modified from Henry's classic extensile approach to the shoulder (Henry, 1973).

Incision (Figure 9.13)

An incision 10 cm long starts 2 cm above the clavicle and passes vertically down, across the tip of the coracoid and distally passes just lateral to the anterior axillary fold.

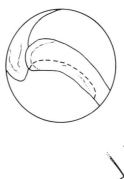

Approach

The cephalic vein is located in the distal deltopectoral groove and dissected upwards, ligating its lateral branches. If bleeding is bothersome the vein may be ligated at the top and bottom of its exposed section. The lateral third of the clavicle is now exposed and the acromioclavicular joint identified using a needle to probe the joint space (Figure 9.14). The periosteum lying over the lateral third of the clavicle is now divided longitudinally retaining the muscular attachments of the deltoid below and the trapezius above. Using an oscillating saw and cutting downwards, the anterior one-third of the thickness of the clavicle is osteotomized from the main part of the bone. The saw cut is brought anteriorly both at the medial attachment of deltoid and just medial to the acromioclavicular joint. The whole of the clavicular attachment of the

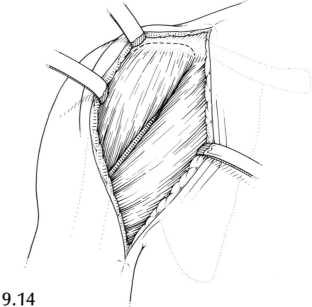

9.14

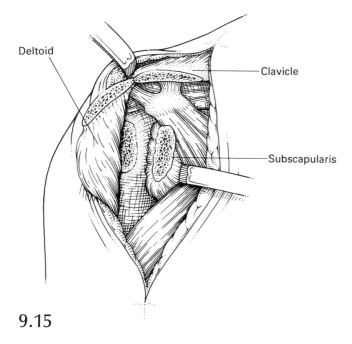

9.15

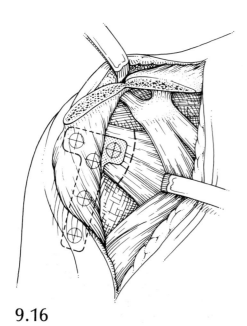

9.16

which is an ill-defined line joining the bicipital groove to the base of the coracoid. Access to the upper humeral shaft is good, providing ideal exposure of the proximal humerus for buttress plating (Figure 9.16). Closure after the operative procedure is carried out by repair of the subscapularis (or lesser tuberosity) with strong (No. 2) non-absorbable sutures, and reattachment of the clavicular osteotomy with three No. 1 absorbable cerclage sutures.

Indications

This approach provides excellent access to the proximal humerus for the surgical reconstruction of fractures of the proximal humerus and for open reduction and fixation of fracture-dislocations of the shoulder. It is also recommended for total shoulder replacement when the glenohumeral joint is stiff and prevents the 40–60 degrees of abduction required for the long anterior deltopectoral approach.

Axillary approach

Access

This approach allows exposure of the front of the shoulder from inferiorly for shoulder stabilization procedures. Good retraction from an assistant is essential.

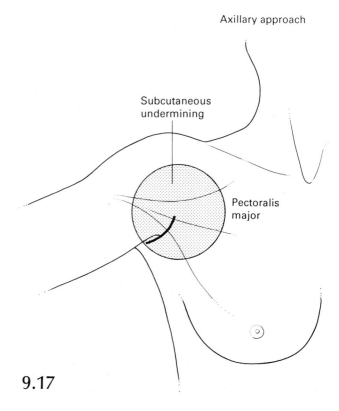

9.17

deltoid now remains firmly attached to the separated bony bar. The split clavicle is gently levered apart using a periosteal elevator and the clavicular head of deltoid can be gently reflected downwards and laterally (Figure 9.15). The rotator cuff may now be exposed by excising the coracoacromial ligament. Access to the glenohumeral joint may be gained by dividing the subscapularis 2 cm from its insertion, or as shown in Figure 9.15 by osteotomizing the lesser tuberosity from the humeral head. The subscapularis tendon is separated from the supraspinatus tendon along the line of the rotator interval

Incision (Figure 9.17)

The incision starts just behind the middle of the anterior axillary fold and is carried posteriorly into the middle of the apex of the axilla. The skin is then widely separated from the underlying soft tissue.

Approach

The lowest centimetre of the pectoralis major tendon is divided vertically for access. Abduction of the arm and retraction of the pectoralis major tendon reveal the subscapularis tendon, the coracobrachialis and the short head of biceps, and in the deepest part of the wound the coracoid process. The pectoralis major tendon should be repaired with strong absorbable sutures at the end of the operation to recreate the normal anterior axillary fold.

Indications

This approach is only indicated in girls and ladies who insist on no visible scar after surgery. Access is poorer than in standard surgical approaches, and the scarring in the axilla can be uncomfortable. It is only recommended for use by surgeons well acquainted with shoulder surgery.

Deltoid-splitting transacromioclavicular joint approach (Ha'Eri and Wiley)

Access

This approach provides a good exposure of the whole of the supraspinatus tendon and, by manipulating the arm, most of the infraspinatus and subscapularis tendons. The whole of the supraspinatus muscle can be exposed by proximal extension of the incision.

Incision (Figure 9.18)

A straight incision, centred on the acromioclavicular joint and approximately 10 cm long is started over the middle of the trapezius proximally, carried downwards and anteriorly over the acromioclavicular joint and then distally passing down in the direction of the fibres of deltoid for a distance of 5 cm from the acromioclavicular joint.

Approach (Figure 9.19)

The incision is deepened proximally by splitting the fibres of the trapezius longitudinally in line with the acromioclavicular joint and likewise distally the deltoid is split for a

distance of 5 cm. If the deltoid is split more distally than 5 cm injury to the anterior branch of the axillary nerve may occur resulting in denervation of the anterior third of deltoid and resultant weakness of the shoulder in flexion. The superior acromioclavicular ligament over the acromioclavicular joint is now divided in line with the joint, the remnant of the meniscus inside the joint is excised and subperiosteal dissection of the periosteum of the lateral clavicle is carried out while maintaining the soft tissue

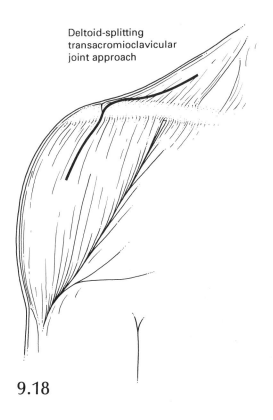

Deltoid-splitting transacromioclavicular joint approach

9.18

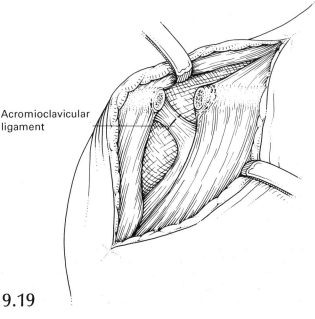

Acromioclavicular ligament

9.19

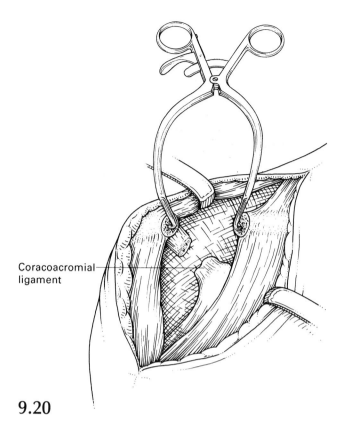

Coracoacromial
ligament

9.20

continuity of the trapezius fibres above with the deltoid
fibres below. This dissection is a little tedious but if carried
out with care results in a very quick and easy closure.
Once the lateral 1 cm of clavicle is exposed a periosteal
elevator is placed under the distal clavicle and using an
oscillating saw the lateral 1 cm of clavicle is removed with a
clean cut in the plane of the acromioclavicular joint.

The acromial side of the incision is now treated in a
similar fashion. The periosteum over the acromion is
carefully dissected using sharp dissection and again
maintaining the continuity of the fibres of the trapezius
above with the deltoid below until the whole of the
anterior acromion is exposed. A Jackson Burrows retractor
can now be placed between the cut surface of the clavicle
medially and the articular surface of the acromial side of
the acromioclavicular joint laterally (Figure 9.20). The
supraspinatus tendon is readily exposed by excision of the
coracoacromial ligament as it passes upwards from the
angle of the coracoid to the undersurface of the acromion.
If rotator cuff surgery is to be carried out excision of the
undersurface of the anterior part of the acromion is
recommended (as described by Neer, 1972), as well as
excision of any spurs arising from the anterior edge of the
acromion, or from the acromial side of the acromioclavicular joint. The whole of the supraspinatus tendon can
now be visualized by manipulating the arm. The subscapularis is brought into view by flexion of the shoulder and
external rotation, while the infraspinatus is visualized by
internal rotation and extension. If mobilization of the
whole of the supraspinatus muscle is required (as part of a

rotator cuff repair), the trapezius muscle is simply split
more proximally and the supraspinatus dissected from the
supraspinous fossa but with care to protect the suprascapular nerve.

Indications

This approach provides an excellent view of the whole of
the supraspinatus and most of the rest of the rotator cuff.
It does not however give access to the most inferior part of
the infraspinatus muscle posteriorly. It is therefore not
appropriate for massive cuff tears where the infraspinatus
is expected to be badly damaged. It allows careful repair
of superior rotator cuff tears and is the best approach to
the subacromial region for the treatment of chronic
impingement lesions.

Transacromial approach (Kessel)

Access

This approach provides a good exposure of the superior
part of the rotator cuff and to the infraspinatus muscle and
tendon posteriorly. It does not allow easy access to the
inferior part of the subscapularis tendon anteriorly.

Incision (Figure 9.21)

The operator's middle finger is placed along the line of the
clavicle, his thumb along the line of the spine of the
scapula and his index finger automatically lies along the
line of the incision. The incision is 10 cm long, with 5 cm
above and 5 cm below the acromion.

Approach (Figure 9.22)

The trapezius and deltoid form a continuous sheet by
blending with the periosteum of the acromion and the
clavicle. By maintaining this continuity during dissection,
there is no opportunity for the muscles to detach or
retract. The muscles are split in the line of their fibres
above and below the acromion. An osteoperiosteal flap is
raised from the acromion, retaining the continuity of the
two muscles. The distal incision in deltoid is limited by the
axillary nerve which has a surface marking at 5 cm distal to
the tip of the acromion where it passes posteriorly around
the humeral neck. The acromion is divided in the coronal
plane using a power saw. (If a decompression of the
anterior part of the rotator cuff is planned this coronal cut
should be carried out only 1 cm posterior to the anterior
tip of the acromion, and the anterior acromial fragment
can then be discarded with little long-term disability.)

A strong self-retaining retractor such as a Jackson
Burrows retractor can now be used to spread the acromial
osteotomy and the related muscles apart (Figure 9.23). At

Transacromial approach

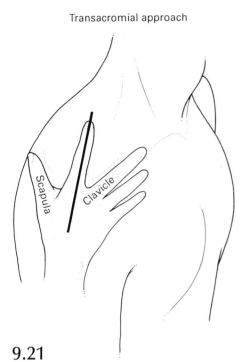

Scapula
Clavicle

9.21

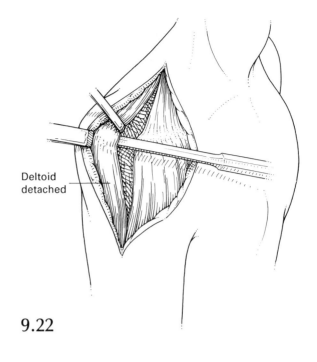

Deltoid
detached

9.22

this stage, either the superior part of the rotator cuff comes into view immediately or the superficial layer of the subacromial bursa may hide it. If the bursa is intact it should be opened along the line of the incision to allow a full inspection of the rotator cuff, which can be manipulated into view by rotating the humerus and moving it into flexion and extension.

During closure the acromion osteotomy is not normally internally fixed. The osteoperiosteal flaps on both sides are brought together and sutured with No. 1 absorbable material. If the anterior part of the acromion has been discarded as part of a decompression procedure, a very careful reconstruction of the anterior part of the deltoid will be necessary. More recently the author has successfully used two 1 mm stainless steel wire inter-osseous sutures to repair the osteotomy.

Indications

The transacromial approach is classically used for the repair of large tears of the rotator cuff. There are two areas which are not readily accessible using this approach – the lower part of subscapularis anteriorly and the surgical neck of the humerus. Thus extensive anterior rotator cuff tears are best approached using the transacromioclavicular joint approach and operations which may require plating of the humeral neck *should not* be carried out using this approach. It is the best approach for the surgical repair of extensive rotator cuff tears affecting the infraspinatus tendon.

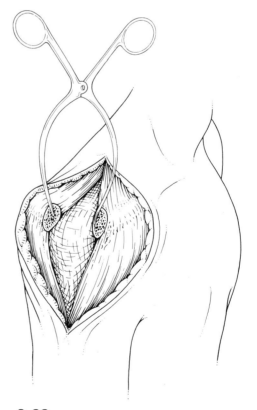

9.23

Posterior approach

Access

This exposure provides access to the posterior aspect of the glenohumeral joint for operations on the infraspinatus tendon or posterior glenoid rim.

Incision (Figure 9.24)

A posterior 'bra-strap' skin incision is recommended.

Approach (Figure 9.25)

The posterior third of the deltoid is detached with periosteum from its origin along the lateral one-third of the spine of the scapula. Care must be taken to avoid dissecting too deeply just inferior to the spine of the scapula as it is very easy to start separating the superior part of infraspinatus from the infraspinous fossa. The posterior belly of deltoid can now be reflected downwards and laterally (Figure 9.26). As this is done the axillary nerve comes into view close to where it emerges from the quadrilateral space. It is usually noted to have two main branches which give a number of muscular fibres to the deep surface of the deltoid. Strong traction *must not* be applied to the detached deltoid as the nerve in this situation is very vulnerable to a traction injury. The infraspinatus and teres minor muscles which lie deep to the deltoid appear to blend together but careful dissection will identify a fascial separation. Access to the posterior aspect of the glenoid is now obtained by identifying the

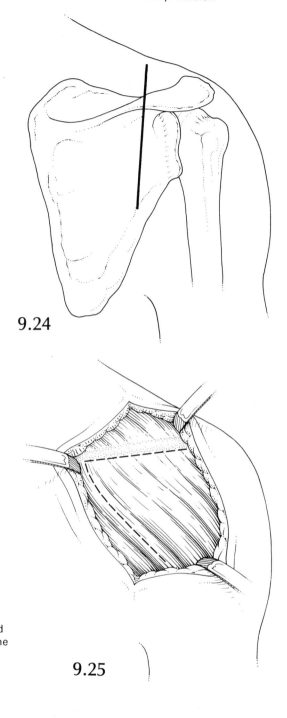

Posterior 'bra-strap' incision

9.24

9.25

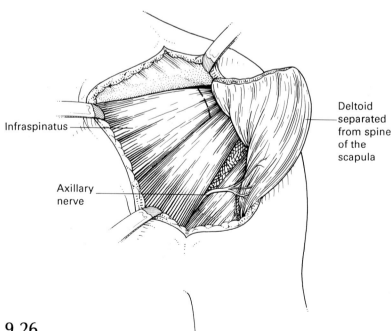

Infraspinatus

Axillary nerve

Deltoid separated from spine of the scapula

9.26

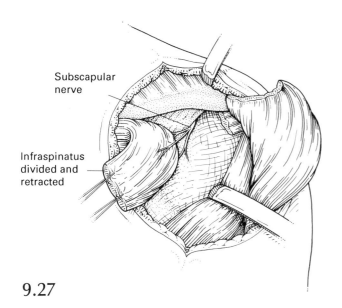

Subscapular
nerve

Infraspinatus
divided and
retracted

9.27

insertion of the infraspinatus and dividing its tendon 1 cm medial to its insertion into the middle area on the greater tuberosity (Figure 9.27). Here again care must be taken to avoid unnecessary dissection around or traction to the suprascapular nerve as it passes downwards around the lateral ridge of the spine of the scapula to innervate the infraspinatus muscle. Full internal rotation of the gleno-humeral joint will now expose the capsule of the joint which is divided vertically to gain access to the posterior glenoid rim. During closure the posterior third of the deltoid is reattached to the spine of the scapula with absorbable sutures passed through drill holes in the scapular spine.

Indications

This approach is used for the surgical correction of recurrent posterior subluxation or dislocation of the shoulder. Probably the most popular operation for this is the glenoid osteotomy and bone graft procedure described by Scott (1967), but a 'reversed' Bankart's operation is also appropriate.

Coronal approach to the acromioclavicular joint

Access

This approach allows a very limited approach to the acromioclavicular joint but because the incision is placed on top of the shoulder is sometimes valuable in a lady for cosmetic reasons.

Incision (Figure 9.28)

The incision is made 2 cm behind and parallel with the lateral one-third of the clavicle.

Approach (Figure 9.29)

The joint is approached through the subcutaneous fat and the acromioclavicular joint may be opened with a coronal incision. A simple closure with absorbable sutures to the deep structures is adequate.

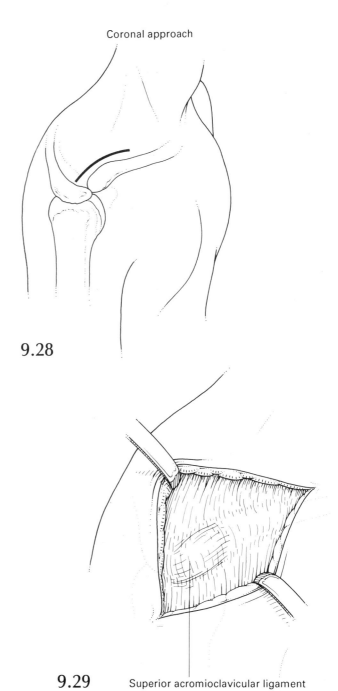

Coronal approach

9.28

9.29   Superior acromioclavicular ligament

Indications

This approach will allow simple meniscectomy of the acromioclavicular joint, excision of the lateral 1 cm of the clavicle for osteoarthritis and open reduction and stabilization of an acromioclavicular joint dislocation.

Parasagittal approach to the acromioclavicular joint

Access

This approach gives generous access to the acromioclavicular joint. It is however important to warn the patient beforehand that the amount of postoperative scarring is unpredictable.

Incision (Figure 9.30)

The incision is made vertically, starting above the clavicle and passing vertically down a distance of about 5 cm over the tip of the coracoid. Experience has indicated that the more medially the incision is placed the less scarring occurs. In ladies it is wise to place the incision so that the scar will lie behind the bra strap.

Approach (Figure 9.31)

The joint is approached through the subcutaneous fat and the acromioclavicular joint is opened with a vertical incision passing above and below in the direction of the fibres of trapezius and deltoid. This approach is essentially a mini version of the transacromioclavicular joint approach described above.

Indications

Excellent access to the acromioclavicular joint for any operation on the joint for arthritis or trauma is provided by this approach. In addition it is the standard approach for a simple subacromial rotator cuff decompression – excision of the coracoacromial ligament and anterior acromioplasty – as recommended by Neer (1972).

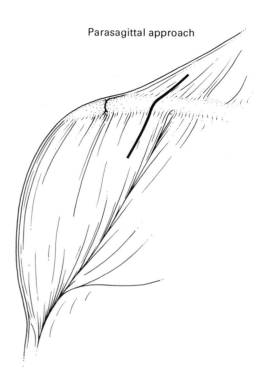

Parasagittal approach

9.30

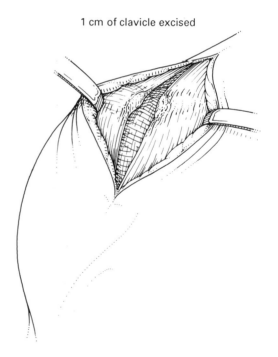

1 cm of clavicle excised

9.31

References

Ha'Eri, G. B. and Wiley, A. M. (1981) Advancement of the supraspinatus muscle in the repair of ruptures of the rotator cuff. *J. Bone Joint Surg.*, **63A**, 232

Henry, A. K. (1973) *Extensive Exposure*, 2nd edn, Churchill Livingstone, Edinburgh, pp. 36–46

Kessel, L. (1982) The transacromial approach for rotator cuff rupture. In *Shoulder Surgery* (eds. I. Bayley and L. Kessel), Springer, Berlin, pp. 39–44

Neer, C. S. II (1972) Anterior acromioplasty for the chronic impingement syndrome in the shoulder. *J. Bone Joint Surg.*, **54A**, 41

Neer, C. S. II, Watson, K. C. and Stanton, F. J. (1982) Recent experience in total shoulder replacement. *J. Bone Joint Surg.*, **64A**, 319

Redfern, T. R., Wallace, W. A. and Beddows, H. (1989) Clavicular osteotomy in shoulder arthroplasty. *Int. Orthop.*, **13**, 61

Scott, D. J. (1967) Treatment of recurrent posterior dislocations of the shoulder by glenoplasty. *J. Bone Joint Surg.*, **49A**, 471

Chapter 10

The humerus

A. E. Freeland and J. L. Hughes

RELEVANT ANATOMY

Superficial cutaneous nerves

The superficial cutaneous nerves communicate where they share a common periphery. Although symptomatic neuromas in the upper arm are unusual, skin incisions should nevertheless be designed to avoid their transection whenever possible.

INTERCOSTOBRACHIAL NERVE (Figure 10.3)

The lateral cutaneous branch of the second intercostal nerve passes into the axilla through the intercostal and serratus anterior muscles to provide sensation to the medial and posterior portion of the upper arm. Frequently, there is a second small contributing branch from the third intercostal nerve. There are often communicating branches between the intercostobrachial and the medial brachial cutaneous nerves.

MEDIAL BRACHIAL CUTANEOUS NERVE (Figures 10.1–10.3)

The medial brachial cutaneous nerve is the smallest branch of the brachial plexus. It arises from the medial cord and crosses the axilla to lie medial to the brachial artery and vein, piercing the deep fascia of the mid-arm to supply its medial sensation. It often communicates with the intercostobrachial nerve.

MEDIAL ANTEBRACHIAL CUTANEOUS NERVE (Figures 10.1–10.3)

The medial antebrachial cutaneous nerve arises from the medial cord of the brachial plexus just distal to the origin of the medial brachial cutaneous nerve. It courses on the medial side of the brachial artery, anterior to the ulnar nerve and anterolateral to the medial brachial cutaneous nerve. High in the arm it gives off its superior branch, which penetrates the deep fascia to supply the anterior skin of the upper arm over the biceps. The main body of the nerve pierces the deep fascia, with the basilic vein, at the middle of the arm and then divides just proximal to the elbow into anterior and posterior branches.

SUPERIOR LATERAL BRACHIAL CUTANEOUS NERVE (Figures 10.2–10.4)

After passing through the quadrilateral space and distributing its motor branches to the deep surfaces of the teres minor and posterior deltoid, the posterior axillary nerve retains only sensory fibres and penetrates the deep fascia at the posterior edge of the deltoid as the superior lateral cutaneous nerve. It then branches to supply the skin over the inferior deltoid and the superior aspect of the long head of the triceps.

POSTERIOR BRACHIAL CUTANEOUS NERVE (Figures 10.2, 10.3)

The posterior brachial cutaneous nerve arises from the radial nerve in the axilla, together with motor branches to the medial triceps. It passes through the axilla to pierce

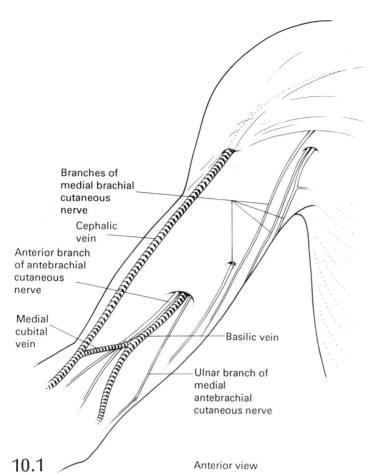

Branches of
medial brachial
cutaneous
nerve

Cephalic
vein

Anterior branch
of antebrachial
cutaneous
nerve

Medial
cubital
vein

Basilic vein

Ulnar branch of
medial
antebrachial
cutaneous
nerve

10.1   Anterior view

the deep fascia and supply skin over the posteromedial
aspect of the upper arm.

INFERIOR LATERAL BRACHIAL CUTANEOUS NERVE
(Figures 10.2, 10.3)

The inferior lateral brachial cutaneous nerve arises from
the radial nerve at the level of the lateral head of the
triceps. It penetrates this muscle and the overlying deep
fascia to proceed anteriorly, lying close to the cephalic
vein. It supplies the posterior and anterolateral portions of
the distal arm.

POSTERIOR ANTEBRACHIAL CUTANEOUS NERVE
(Figures 10.2, 10.3)

The posterior antebrachial cutaneous nerve may arise
from the radial nerve, either from a common trunk with
the inferior lateral brachial cutaneous nerve, or as a
separate branch just distal and inferior to it. It penetrates
the lateral head of the triceps just before the radial nerve
passes through the lateral intermuscular septum. It then
courses distally, penetrating the brachial fascia in the arm
and goes posterior to the lateral humeral epicondyle. It
innervates the distal posterior portion of the arm and part
of the back of the forearm (Figure 12.1(b)).

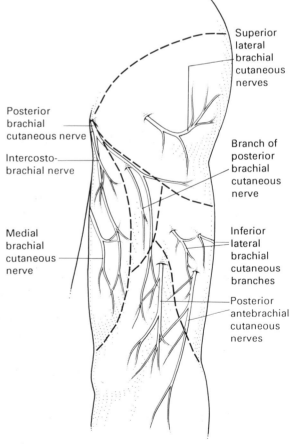

Posterior
brachial
cutaneous nerve

Intercosto-
brachial nerve

Medial
brachial
cutaneous
nerve

Superior
lateral
brachial
cutaneous
nerves

Branch of
posterior
brachial
cutaneous
nerve

Inferior
lateral
brachial
cutaneous
branches

Posterior
antebrachial
cutaneous
nerves

10.2   Posterior view

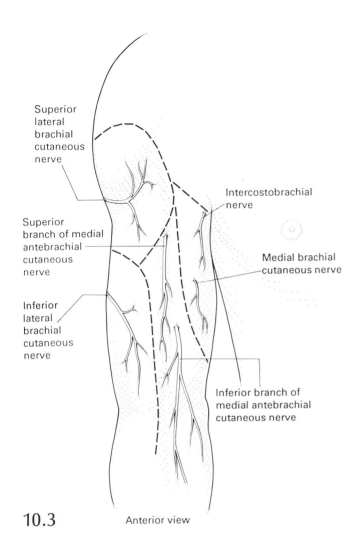

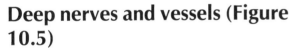

10.3   Anterior view

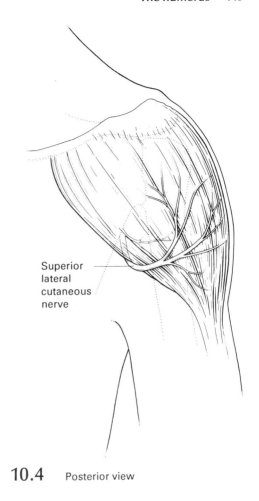

10.4   Posterior view

Deep nerves and vessels (Figure 10.5)

All the muscles of the upper arm are innervated by the musculocutaneous and radial nerves. The median and ulnar nerves pass through the upper arm to reach the muscles of the forearm and hand. The median nerve enters the arm lateral to the brachial artery, crossing it anteriorly at the level of the insertion of coracobrachialis and then descends medial to the artery to enter the antecubital fossa. The ulnar nerve enters the arm medial to the brachial artery and vein and posterior to the medial antebrachial cutaneous nerve. At the mid-arm level, it diverges posteriorly, piercing the medial intermuscular septum and then continues with the superior ulnar collateral artery, on the deep surface of the medial head of triceps, to the posterior aspect of the medial epicondyle.

MUSCULOCUTANEOUS NERVE (Figure 10.6)

Just below the inferior border of the pectoralis minor, the musculocutaneous nerve enters the arm, after first giving

off branches to supply the coracobrachialis, then passing through this muscle. Just as it leaves the coracobrachialis it branches to supply both heads of the biceps muscle, when the nerve lies between the biceps and the brachialis. It then branches at the mid-arm level to supply the brachialis, after which it continues as a purely sensory nerve in the lower arm, as the lateral antebrachial cutaneous nerve.

RADIAL NERVE (Figure 10.7)

The radial nerve is the largest branch of the brachial plexus and is a continuation of the posterior cord. It enters the proximal arm posterior to the brachial artery and anterior to the long head of the triceps. It then descends obliquely and laterally and arrives in the posterior arm with the profunda brachii artery by passing through the triangular space bounded superiorly by the inferior border of the teres major, medially by the lateral border of the long head of the triceps and laterally by the medial border of the medial head of the triceps. It then takes a spiral course down the arm close to the humerus and parallel and just superior to the profunda brachii artery. It lies a finger's breadth below the insertion of the deltoid and courses just distal to the spiral groove lying on the proximal portion of the origin of the medial head of

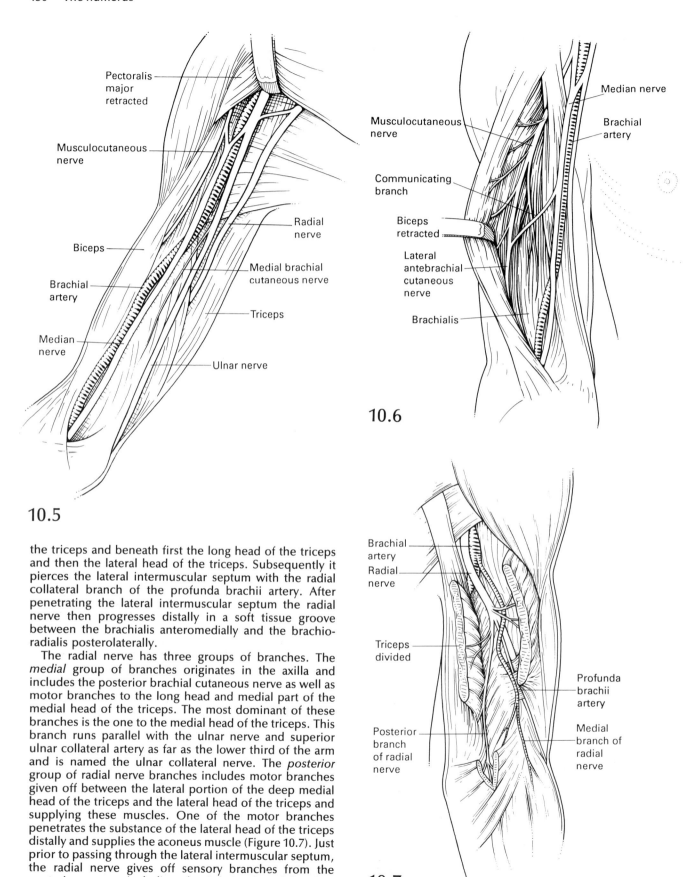

Pectoralis major retracted

Musculocutaneous nerve

Biceps

Brachial artery

Median nerve

Radial nerve

Medial brachial cutaneous nerve

Triceps

Ulnar nerve

10.5

Musculocutaneous nerve

Communicating branch

Biceps retracted

Lateral antebrachial cutaneous nerve

Brachialis

Median nerve

Brachial artery

10.6

Brachial artery

Radial nerve

Triceps divided

Posterior branch of radial nerve

Profunda brachii artery

Medial branch of radial nerve

10.7

the triceps and beneath first the long head of the triceps and then the lateral head of the triceps. Subsequently it pierces the lateral intermuscular septum with the radial collateral branch of the profunda brachii artery. After penetrating the lateral intermuscular septum the radial nerve then progresses distally in a soft tissue groove between the brachialis anteromedially and the brachio-radialis posterolaterally.

The radial nerve has three groups of branches. The *medial* group of branches originates in the axilla and includes the posterior brachial cutaneous nerve as well as motor branches to the long head and medial part of the medial head of the triceps. The most dominant of these branches is the one to the medial head of the triceps. This branch runs parallel with the ulnar nerve and superior ulnar collateral artery as far as the lower third of the arm and is named the ulnar collateral nerve. The *posterior* group of radial nerve branches includes motor branches given off between the lateral portion of the deep medial head of the triceps and the lateral head of the triceps and supplying these muscles. One of the motor branches penetrates the substance of the lateral head of the triceps distally and supplies the aconeus muscle (Figure 10.7). Just prior to passing through the lateral intermuscular septum, the radial nerve gives off sensory branches from the posterior group, including the inferior lateral brachial cutaneous nerve and the posterior antebrachial cutaneous nerve (Figure 10.2). These two sensory branches may arise from a common trunk. After piercing the lateral intermuscular septum, the radial nerve gives off its lateral group of branches, including one or more which may penetrate and sometimes supply the posterolateral aspect of the brachialis muscle and then continue through it to supply the elbow joint. Further distally, motor branches supply first the brachioradialis and then the extensor carpi radialis longus muscles.

BRACHIAL ARTERY (Figure 10.5)

The brachial artery begins as a continuation of the axillary artery at the inferior border of the teres major muscle. It lies anterior to the long head of the triceps, then, in turn, on the deep surface of the medial head, the insertion of the coracobrachialis and finally the brachialis muscle. It passes from the medial side of the humerus proximally to the mid-point anteriorly at the elbow. The biceps lies anterolaterally. Medially, the brachial artery is covered by skin, subcutaneous fat and deep fascia. There are two brachial veins, one medial and one lateral to the brachial artery. The relationships of the major nerves to the brachial artery are described above.

The brachial artery gives off several branches including the profunda brachii artery, the nutrient artery of the humerus, the superior and inferior ulnar collateral arteries and muscular branches in the arm.

The *profunda brachii artery* is the largest branch of the brachial artery and arises from the posteromedial side of the brachial artery in the upper arm. It then passes downwards and laterally behind the brachial artery, to run parallel with the radial nerve, just inferior to the spiral groove, first deep to the long head and then the lateral head of the triceps and on top of the deep medial triceps head (Figure 10.7). As it approaches the lateral intermuscular septum it branches into the middle collateral artery which supplies the medial head of the triceps and the radial collateral artery which continues with the radial nerve through the remainder of its course in the arm supplying adjacent muscles.

CEPHALIC VEIN (Figure 10.8)

The cephalic vein ascends subcutaneously in the arm, superficial to the groove between the brachioradialis and the lateral edge of the biceps, until it courses medially in the upper arm to lie in the deltopectoral interval.

BASILIC VEIN (Figure 10.8)

The basilic vein runs subcutaneously, medial to the biceps and perforates the deep fascia a little below the middle of the upper arm, accompanied by the medial antebrachial cutaneous nerve. It enters the anterior compartment to lie medial to both the brachial artery and medial brachial vein, until it reaches the inferior border of the teres major where it joins with the medial brachial vein to become the axillary vein.

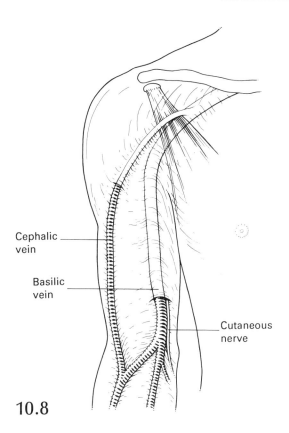

Cephalic vein

Basilic vein

Cutaneous nerve

10.8

Fascia and muscles of the arm

DEEP BRACHIAL FASCIA

Proximally, the deep brachial fascia of the arm is continuous with that of the deltoid muscle laterally and with that of the pectoralis major and latissimus dorsi muscles medially. Distally, it fastens to the epicondyles of the humerus and the olecranon and is continuous with the antebrachial fascia. It forms a loose sheath for the muscles of the arm and invests them with septa, the strongest of which are the medial and lateral intermuscular septa that divide the arm into anterior and posterior compartments.

Anterior compartment of the arm (Figures 10.5, 10.6, 10.8)

The anterior compartment of the arm contains the brachial artery, the brachial and basilic veins, the median nerve, the proximal half of the ulnar nerve, the biceps, brachialis, brachioradialis and extensor carpi radialis longus.

Biceps brachii

The biceps brachii muscle originates from a short head lateral to, and confluent with, the origin of the coracobrachialis at the apex of the coracoid process and from a long head at the superior glenoid tubercle. It is the most anterior muscle in the arm, innervated by the musculocutaneous nerve, and inserts both on the bicipital tuberosity of the radius and medially, via the bicipital aponeurosis, into the deep fascia of the proximal forearm. The biceps is an elbow flexor, a forearm supinator and an accessory stabilizer and flexor of the shoulder.

Coracobrachialis muscle

The coracobrachialis originates from the tip of the coracoid process in common with the short head of the biceps. It is innervated by the musculocutaneous nerve, inserts in the medial humeral shaft and adducts and flexes the arm, while contributing to shoulder stability.

Brachialis muscle

The brachialis originates from the anterior aspect of the lower half of the humerus. It is innervated by the musculocutaneous nerve and, to a much lesser extent, laterally by one or more branches of the radial nerve. It inserts on the tuberosity of the ulna and the coronoid process, acting as an elbow flexor.

Brachioradialis muscle

The brachioradialis arises from the upper two-thirds of the lateral supracondylar ridge of the humerus and from the anterior surface of the lateral intermuscular septum. It is supplied by the radial nerve, attaches to the base of the styloid process of the radius and flexes the elbow.

Extensor carpi radialis longus muscle

The extensor carpi radialis longus muscle is overlapped by the brachioradialis and arises from the lower third of the lateral supracondylar ridge of the humerus, the front of the lateral intermuscular septum and the common tendon of origin of the forearm extensors. It is supplied by the radial nerve, attaches to the dorsal base of the second metacarpal and extends and radially deviates the wrist.

Posterior compartment of the arm (Figure 10.7)

The posterior compartment of the arm contains the triceps, the radial nerve, the profunda brachii artery and the inferior half of the ulnar nerve.

Triceps muscle

The triceps muscle arises from three heads: the long head originates from the infraglenoid tubercle of the scapula; the lateral head arises from a narrow ridge on the posterior shaft of the humerus and from the lateral

intermuscular septum; the deep medial head arises from the posterior humerus below the spiral groove and from the medial and lateral intermuscular septa. It is innervated by the radial nerve, inserts by a common tendon into the olecranon and extends the elbow.

SURGICAL APPROACHES

- Posterior triceps splitting (Henry, 1924)
- Proximal anterolateral (Thompson, 1918 and Henry, 1973)
- Distal anterolateral

Posterior triceps splitting approach (Henry)

Access

This approach provides access to the middle two-thirds of the posterior humeral shaft and to the radial nerve at the same level.

Position

The patient may be positioned either prone with the arm abducted, resting on an adjacent side-table and with the elbow flexed over the end of the side-table, or supine with the arm flexed, adducted and internally rotated at the shoulder.

Incision

A mid-line posterior longitudinal incision is made parallel to the long axis of the humerus from the posterior border of the deltoid, 5 cm inferior to the acromial angle, to the level of the olecranon fossa (Figure 10.9(a)).

Approach

The underlying superficial and deep fasciae are incised in line with the incision. The V-shaped interval between the long and lateral heads of the triceps is identified proximally (Figure 10.9(b)), lifted with a finger and split to the distal extent of the incision (Figure 10.9(c)). The neurovascular bundle containing the radial nerve and profunda brachii artery will be seen coursing obliquely laterally and distally along the superior border of the deep medial head of the triceps just below the spiral groove (Figure 10.9(d)). Take care to identify and protect this neurovascular bundle and its branches. Particular care

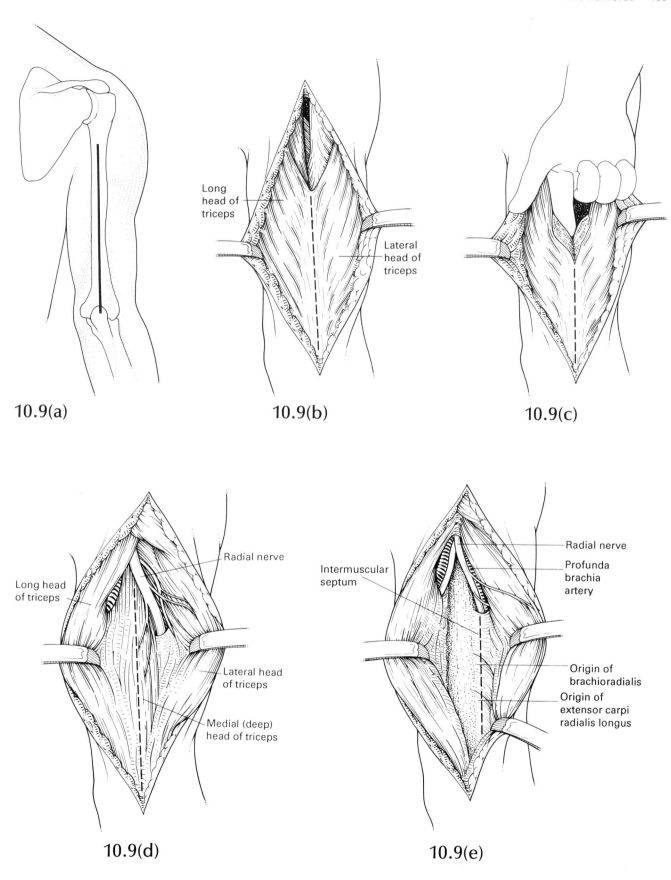

10.9(a)

10.9(b)

Long
head of
triceps

Lateral
head of
triceps

10.9(c)

10.9(d)

Long head
of triceps

Radial nerve

Lateral head
of triceps

Medial (deep)
head of triceps

10.9(e)

Intermuscular
septum

Radial nerve

Profunda
brachia
artery

Origin of
brachioradialis

Origin of
extensor carpi
radialis longus

should be taken to protect the nerve to the lateral head of the triceps, which runs a more transverse course than its parent radial nerve. The deep medial head of the triceps is split in the mid-line and the humerus is exposed subperiosteally (Figures 10.9(d),(e)). This incision will not damage the nerve supply to the deep medial head if care is taken to avoid injury of the ulnar collateral nerve which supplies its inner half and of those branches to its outer half given off by the radial nerve after it passes the medial border of the lateral head of the triceps. The ulnar nerve lies deep to the long head of the triceps so that, distally, the incision of the deep medial head of the triceps should remain close to the medial border of the lateral head, in order to avoid damage to the ulnar nerve and superior ulnar collateral artery after they pierce the medial intermuscular septum. When the outer half of the deep medial head of the triceps is fully raised from the back of the humerus, the lateral intermuscular septum comes into view along with the origins of the brachioradialis and extensor carpi radialis longus. These structures can be divided to expose the radial nerve as it passes anteriorly and laterally down the middle two-thirds of the arm (Figure 10.9(e)).

Indications

This incision is particularly useful for access to lesions of the middle two-thirds of the humeral shaft, as well as for repair or reconstruction of fractures in the same region. The radial nerve may also be approached at these levels when indicated.

Proximal anterolateral approach (Thompson and Henry)

Access

This approach gives access to the proximal and middle thirds of the humeral shaft. The incision is extensile proximally with the anterior deltopectoral approach to the shoulder, so that the entire proximal humerus may be exposed.

Position

The patient is positioned supine. The arm is placed on an arm board that is located so that its long axis is parallel to the long axis of the operating table. The arm is then rested on this support so that the shoulder may be abducted, adducted or internally or externally rotated.

Incision

The incision starts proximally along the anterior margin of the deltoid, 5 cm below the acromion process. When the

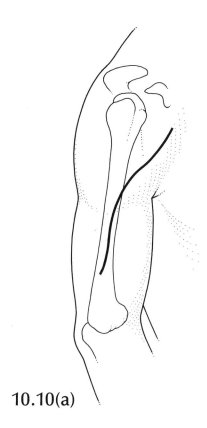

10.10(a)

incision reaches the insertion of the deltoid it is curved to run distally, parallel to the lateral border of the biceps. It ends 7.5 cm above the elbow joint, just proximal to the origin of the brachioradialis muscle (Figure 10.10(a)).

Approach

The superficial and deep fasciae are divided in line with the incision. The cephalic vein is protected and retracted medially (if necessary, dividing any tributaries joining it from the deltoid), as the interval between the deltoid and the pectoralis major muscles is developed. Distal to the insertion of the deltoid muscle, the brachialis is split longitudinally along a line marking the junction of its lateral third and medial two-thirds (Figure 10.10(b)). The humerus is exposed by extraperiosteal or subperiosteal dissection (Figure 10.10(c)). Retraction is easier when the elbow is flexed to relax the brachialis muscle. The lateral third of the brachialis usually protects the radial nerve, but if there is any question, the radial nerve should be identified and exposed sufficiently so that it can be protected.

Indications

This incision may be used for removal of benign or malignant tumours and for infections of the proximal two-thirds of the humeral shaft. It is used also for repair or reconstruction of fractures in the same region.

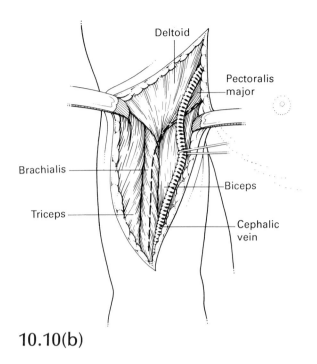

10.10(b)

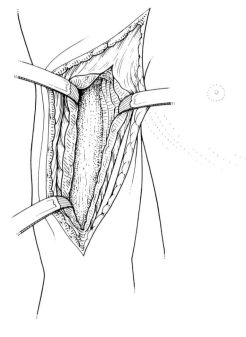

Humerus exposed

10.10(c)

Distal anterolateral approach

Access

This approach exposes the junction of the middle and distal thirds of the humeral shaft and the radial nerve at the same level. The incision is extensile with the proximal anterolateral incision of the arm described above (see p. 154) and distally with the anterolateral incision of the forearm (see p. 185).

Incision

The incision begins proximally at the origin of the brachioradialis muscle, about 10 cm above the elbow, and extends distally in the groove between the biceps and the brachioradialis, to end in the antecubital region (Figure 10.11(a)).

Approach

The subcutaneous and deep fasciae are divided in line with the incision. The interval between the brachioradialis and brachialis proximally and the brachioradialis and biceps distally, is developed so that the brachioradialis may be retracted laterally and the brachialis and biceps medially (Figure 10.11(b)). The radial nerve is located deep in the incision along the anterolateral aspect of the humerus and is identified proximally between the brachioradialis and brachialis muscles. It gives branches to the brachioradialis muscle at this level. The radial nerve can either be left undisturbed or may be mobilized and retracted laterally to safeguard it from injury. The lateral margin of the brachialis is separated from the radial nerve and retracted medially to expose the periosteum of the humerus. The periosteum is incised in line with the lateral margin of the brachialis (Figure 10.11(c)) and the junction of the middle and distal thirds of the humerus exposed subperiosteally (Figure 10.11(d)).

Indications

This incision is used for the surgery of tumours or infection of the junction of the middle and distal thirds of the humeral shaft. It may be used also for repair or reconstruction of fractures of this same region. The radial nerve may also be approached in this region.

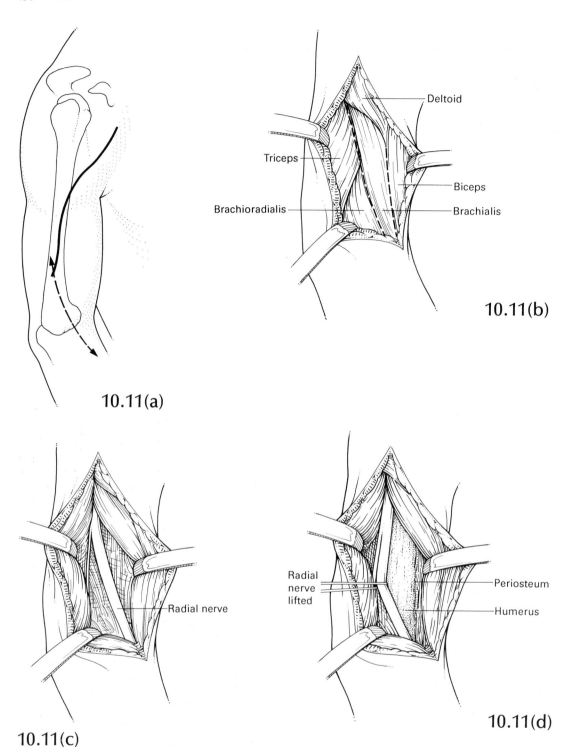

10.11(a)

10.11(b)

Deltoid

Triceps

Brachioradialis

Biceps

Brachialis

10.11(c)

Radial nerve

10.11(d)

Radial
nerve
lifted

Periosteum

Humerus

References

Henry, A. K. (1924–25) Exposure of the humerus and femoral
  shaft. *Br. J. Surg.*, **12**, 84
Henry, A. K. (1973) *Extensile Exposure*, 2nd edn, Churchill
  Livingstone, Edinburgh
Thompson, J. E. (1918) Anatomical methods of approach in
  operations on the long bones of the extremities. *Ann. Surg.*,
  65, 309

Further reading

Crenshaw, A. H. (1980) Surgical approaches. In *Campbell's
  Operative Orthopedics*, 6th edn (eds A. S. Edmonson and A. H.
  Crenshaw), C. V. Mosby, St Louis
Ip, M. D. and Chang, K. S. F. (1968) A study on the radial supply of
  the human brachialis muscle. *Anat. Rec.*, **162**, 363
Pineiro, S. J. and Esperne, P. (1939) Surgical anatomy of the arm:
  paths of approach to the humerus. *Rev. Surg., Buenos Aires*, 18

Chapter 11

The elbow

A. E. Freeland and J. L. Hughes

RELEVANT ANATOMY

LATERAL ANTEBRACHIAL CUTANEOUS NERVE (Figure 11.1(a),(b))

The remaining sensory portion of the musculocutaneous nerve penetrates the deep fascia near the lateral border of the biceps tendon. It lies deep to and between the cephalic and accessory cephalic veins and supplies the lower anterolateral portion of the elbow region (Figure 11.1(b)).

POSTERIOR ANTEBRACHIAL CUTANEOUS NERVE (Figure 11.1(c))

The posterior antebrachial cutaneous nerve is part of the posterior group of radial nerve branches that arise in the region of the lateral head of the triceps (see p. 148). It arises in common with the inferior lateral brachial cutaneous nerve. It descends along the posterolateral aspect of the arm to supply skin over the posterior and posterolateral surfaces of the region.

ANTECUBITAL FOSSA (Figure 11.2(a),(b))

The antecubital fossa is triangular and lies in front of the elbow joint. Its base is proximal and is formed by a hypothetical line between the two humeral epicondyles. The sides are formed by the medial margin of the brachioradialis laterally and the lateral border of the pronator teres medially, converging distally to meet at the apex. The floor is composed of the brachialis and the supinator. Anteriorly, in sequence, lie the skin, subcutaneous fascia, containing cutaneous nerves and subcutaneous veins (including the median antecubital vein), and the deep fascia reinforced by the bicipital aponeurosis (Figure 11.2(a)). The space contains, from medial to lateral beneath the bicipital aponeurosis and deep fascia, first the median nerve, secondly, the brachial artery lying in the middle of the fossa and, thirdly, the biceps tendon (mnemonic MAT). Near the apex of the antecubital fossa the brachial artery divides into its radial and ulnar branches, the latter being posterior to, and separated by, the ulnar head of pronator teres from the median nerve. Laterally, the radial nerve lies just adjacent to the antecubital fossa between the brachioradialis and the supinator (Figure 11.2(b)).

SUPRACONDYLAR PROCESS AND THE LIGAMENT OF STRUTHERS (Figure 11.2(c))

The supracondylar process is an anteromedial bony spur that projects from the lower humerus in 1% of all upper extremities. The ligament of Struthers extends from the tip of the supracondylar process to the junction of the medial epicondyle and the humeral metaphysis. The supracondylar process and the ligament of Struthers are anterior to the medial intermuscular septum. The median nerve and brachial artery pass deep to these structures and occasionally an entrapment syndrome results.

Deep nerves and vessels

It is noteworthy that the three major peripheral nerves of the upper extremity ordinarily leave the elbow region and

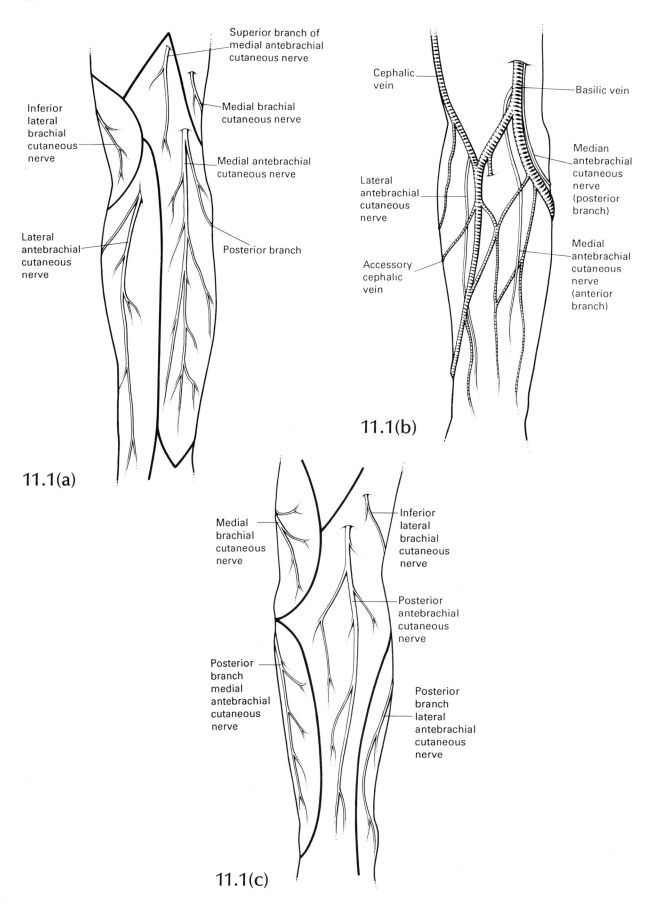

Superior branch of
medial antebrachial
cutaneous nerve

Medial brachial
cutaneous nerve

Medial antebrachial
cutaneous nerve

Posterior branch

Inferior
lateral
brachial
cutaneous
nerve

Lateral
antebrachial
cutaneous
nerve

11.1(a)

Cephalic
vein

Basilic vein

Lateral
antebrachial
cutaneous
nerve

Accessory
cephalic
vein

Median
antebrachial
cutaneous
nerve
(posterior
branch)

Medial
antebrachial
cutaneous
nerve
(anterior
branch)

11.1(b)

Medial
brachial
cutaneous
nerve

Inferior
lateral
brachial
cutaneous
nerve

Posterior
antebrachial
cutaneous
nerve

Posterior
branch
medial
antebrachial
cutaneous
nerve

Posterior
branch
lateral
antebrachial
cutaneous
nerve

11.1(c)

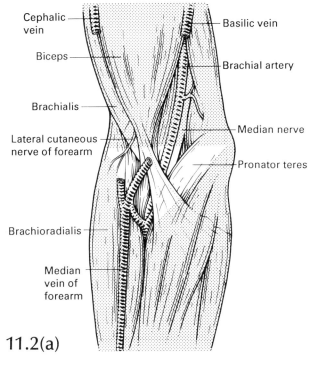

11.2(a)

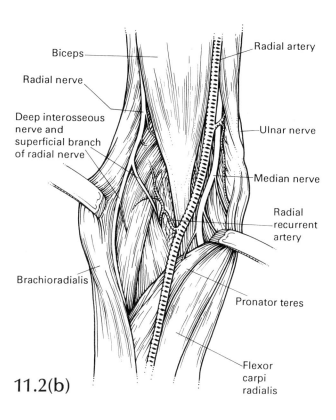

11.2(b)

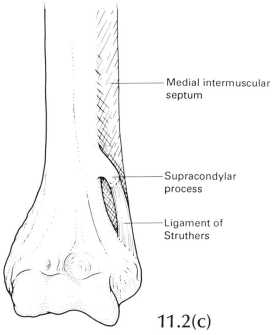

11.2(c)

enter the forearm between two muscular heads; the median nerve between the two heads of pronator teres, the ulnar nerve between the two heads of the flexor carpi ulnaris and the posterior interosseous branch of the radial nerve between the two heads of the supinator.

MEDIAN NERVE (Figure 11.2(a),(b))

The median nerve enters the antecubital fossa medial to the brachial artery. It may give off a muscular branch to the pronator teres as high as 7 cm above the elbow joint but more frequently this branch leaves the main nerve trunk 1–2 cm below the elbow joint. It then courses somewhat obliquely from medial to lateral across the antecubital space beneath the lacertus fibrosus and on top of the brachialis muscle. Articular branches are distributed to the elbow joint and the proximal radio-ulnar joint. The median nerve crosses over the ulnar artery from medial to lateral as it enters between the superficial and deep heads of the pronator teres, the deep head separating it from the ulnar artery. The remaining branches of the median nerve to the forearm muscles are highly variable in the distal half of the antecubital fossa and proximal forearm and will be discussed in the chapter on the forearm (see Chapter 12).

RADIAL NERVE (Figure 11.2(b))

After the radial nerve and the radial collateral branch of the profunda brachii artery pass forwards through the lateral intermuscular septum, they pass anterior to the lateral humeral epicondyle behind the lateral edge of the brachialis muscle and between this muscle and the brachioradialis. The radial nerve then gives off its lateral branches. First, it gives off a branch to the brachialis muscle which terminates anteriorly as an articular branch to the elbow joint. Distal to this, but above the elbow joint, it gives off branches first to the brachioradialis and then to the extensor carpi radialis longus. The branch to the extensor carpi radialis brevis may occasionally come off the radial nerve at the elbow joint before the radial nerve divides into its superficial sensory and deep motor branches, but more frequently it is the first branch of the posterior interosseous nerve. The radial nerve divides into its superficial sensory and posterior interosseous motor branches at or below the epicondylar level of the elbow. The superficial branch of the radial nerve, which is entirely sensory, descends under the cover of the brachioradialis to leave the region of the elbow. The deep posterior interosseous branch leaves the elbow region between the two heads of the supinator muscle.

ULNAR NERVE (Figure 11.3)

After the ulnar nerve pierces the medial intermuscular septum, it slopes medially accompanied by the superior ulnar collateral artery on the medial head of the triceps to reach its groove on the dorsum of the medial humeral epicondyle where it is secured by overlying retinaculum (the cubital tunnel). As it leaves its groove it lies on the posterior oblique ulnar collateral ligament. It may give off its articular branches here or higher. Then one or more branches are given off to the flexor carpi ulnaris, prior to passing between the two muscular heads, followed by one or more branches to the ulnar half of the flexor digitorum profundus.

BRACHIAL ARTERY AND COLLATERAL CIRCULATION TO THE ELBOW (Figures 11.2(a),(b), 11.4)

The brachial artery lies medial to the biceps as it enters then passes through the antecubital fossa, anterior to the brachialis and under the lacertus fibrosus. The median nerve lies medial to it in the antecubital fossa. The brachial artery terminates in the antecubital fossa about 1 cm below the elbow joint level by dividing into the radial and ulnar arteries. In the antecubital fossa, the radial artery is the smaller, but more direct, continuation of the brachial artery and courses laterally anterior to the biceps tendon and supinator, and gives off first the radial recurrent artery

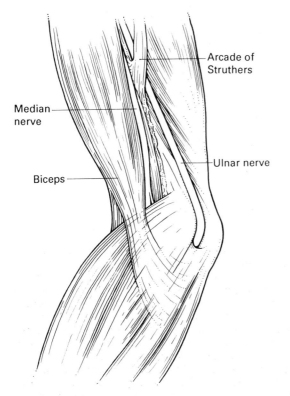

11.3(a)

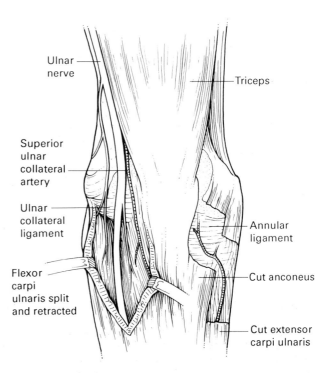

11.3(b)

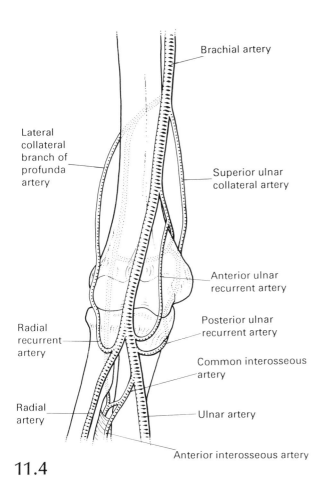

11.4

and then a leash of unnamed muscular branches to the brachioradialis and extensor carpi radialis longus and brevis muscles anteriorly. The radial recurrent artery curves laterally and ascends adjacent to the radial nerve between the brachialis and the brachioradialis to anastomose with the radial collateral branch of the profunda brachii artery.

The ulnar artery runs downwards and medially and leaves the antecubital fossa under the deep ulnar head of pronator teres, which separates it from the median nerve. It then rejoins the median nerve between the two heads of the flexor digitorum superficialis in the proximal forearm and gives off branches critical to the collateral circulation of the elbow.

Muscles

ANCONEUS (Figure 11.5)

The triangular anconeus arises from the posterior surface of the lateral epicondyle, covers the posterior aspect of the annular ligament and inserts into the lateral aspect of the olecranon and the upper quarter of the posterior ulnar shaft. It is innervated by a long branch from the posterior

group of radial branches (see Chapter 10) that reaches it through the medial head of the triceps. It assists elbow extension and stabilizes the ulna during pronation. It is the primary abductor of the forearm.

OTHER MUSCLES

The humeral head of the pronator teres originates on the inferior extent of the medial supracondylar ridge proximal to the common flexor origin from the medial epicondyle (Figure 11.2(a),(b)). The three heads of the triceps converge to insert into an aponeurosis over the anconeus and a tendon into the olecranon. The brachioradialis originates high on the lateral supracondylar ridge with the radial wrist extensors below it on the inferior half of the ridge (Figure 11.2(b)). The common extensor origin is from the lateral epicondyle.

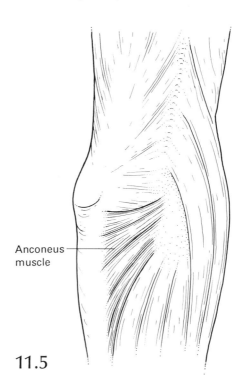

11.5

The elbow joint

The elbow joint is a compound synovial joint comprising the humero-ulnar joint (between the trochlea of the humerus and the trochlear notch of the ulna) and the radiohumeral joint (between the capitellum of the humerus and the head of the radius). The cubital articulation includes both the compound elbow joint and the superior radioulnar joint. Flexion and extension occur at the humero-ulnar and radiohumeral joints, while rotation of the forearm occurs at the radiohumeral and radio-ulnar joints. The elbow joint is innervated by the musculocutaneous, radial, median and ulnar nerves, adhering to the basic rule that a joint is innervated by the nerves that cross it.

Ligaments

ULNAR COLLATERAL LIGAMENT COMPLEX (Figure 11.6(a))

The ulnar collateral ligament complex is a thick triangular ligament attached at its apex to the medial humeral epicondyle and fanning to attach at its base to the medial side of the olecranon. It consists of three parts. The anterior part is triangular, arising at its apex from the anterior aspect of the medial humeral epicondyle and attaching to a tubercle on the superomedial aspect of the coronoid process of the olecranon. The posterior band of the ulnar collateral ligament is also triangular, arising at its apex from the postero-inferior aspect of the medial humeral epicondyle, spreading distally to attach to the medial border of the olecranon. The thinner intermediate portion arises and attaches between the anterior and posterior components. The oblique band of the ulnar collateral ligament consists of a parallel thickening of capsular fibres between the insertions of the anterior and posterior ulnar collateral ligaments.

RADIAL COLLATERAL LIGAMENT (Figure 11.6(b))

The radial collateral ligament of the elbow joint originates at the inferior lateral humeral epicondyle and fans distally to insert into the annular ligament and the proximal supinator crest of the ulna.

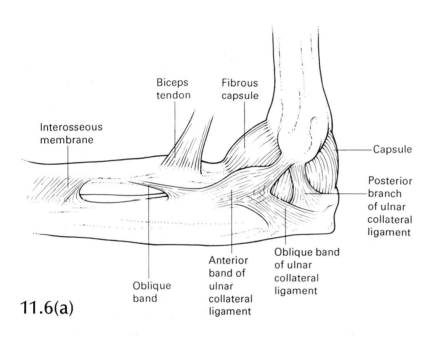

11.6(a)

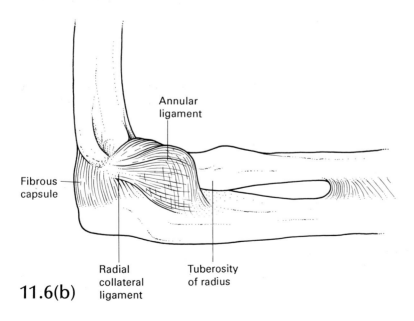

11.6(b)

ANNULAR LIGAMENT

The annular ligament extends from the anterior to the posterior margin of the radial notch, encircling and containing the radial head within this notch.

QUADRATE LIGAMENT

The quadrate ligament extends between the lateral side of the proximal ulna just distal to the radial notch and the neck of the radius just distal to the articular margin in line with the bicipital tuberosity. It contributes to the stability of the proximal radio-ulnar joint, particularly in the extremes of pronation and supination (Spinner and Kaplan, 1970).

SURGICAL APPROACHES

- Posterior (Campbell, Van Gorder)
- Posterior longitudinal with or without osteotomy of olecranon
- Posterior – transolecranon 'U' (MacAusland)
- Lateral
- Posterolateral (Kocher)
- Anterior (Pheasant)
- Medial (Molesworth, Campbell, Learmouth)
- Posterior – olecranon and proximal ulna

Posterior approach (Campbell, Van Gorder)

Access

This approach provides access to the distal humerus including its articular surface.

Position

The patient may be positioned prone with the elbow flexed over a well-padded arm board, or supine with the shoulder adducted and the elbow flexed across the torso, stabilized by an assistant holding the wrist and forearm.

Incision

The incision is made in the posterior mid-line, starting 15 cm above the olecranon and extending it downwards to 3 cm distal to the tip of the olecranon. The distal end of the incision should be curved lateral to the olecranon in order to avoid this bony prominence (Figure 11.7(a)).

Approach

Expose the lower portion of the triceps muscle and its tendon of insertion and expansions. Identify, expose and protect the ulnar nerve, using a moist tape. Cut the triceps tendon in the shape of a tongue: the apex of this tongue should be 10 cm above the olecranon and the distal base should extend to the outer border of the humeral condyles at the joint line (Figure 11.7(b)). The apex of the tongue will consist of fascia only, the mid-portion will consist of fascia and muscle and the base of the tongue at the joint line will include the full thickness of the triceps muscle and tendon. After reflecting the tongue, a longitudinal, mid-line incision is made through the remaining muscle down to the bone. Dissection to either side exposes the posterior surface of the lower end of the humerus and the joint (Figure 11.7(c)).

Indications

This approach is used to restore unreduced elbow dislocations and to correct extension contractures of the elbow. It is also an excellent approach for open reduction and internal fixation of supracondylar fractures in children and adults. In addition, it is a superior approach for corrective osteotomy at the supracondylar level of the humerus and for treating delayed or non-unions at this level. This approach may be used for open reduction and internal fixation of comminuted intra-articular fractures of the distal humerus, but those approaches that allow removal of the olecranon provide better access for joint restoration in the adult and also permit immediate joint motion. Arthroplasty can be performed utilizing this approach and heterotopic bone may be resected.

Posterior longitudinal approach with or without osteotomy of the olecranon

Access

This approach provides access to the triceps tendon, the distal humerus including its articular surface, the elbow joint, the radial head and the olecranon.

Position

The patient may be positioned as for the posterior approach.

Incision

The incision starts from the posterior mid-line of the arm 10 cm above the tip of the olecranon and is directed

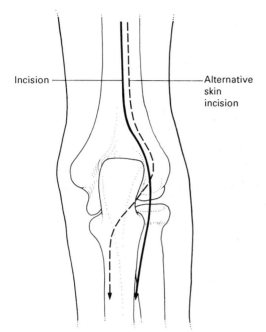

11.7(a)

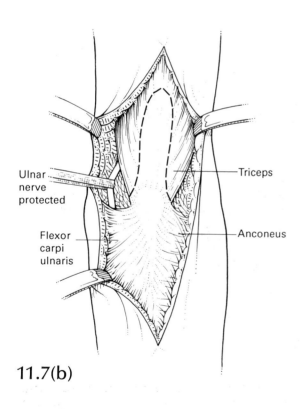

Ulnar
nerve
protected

Flexor
carpi
ulnaris

Triceps

Anconeus

11.7(b)

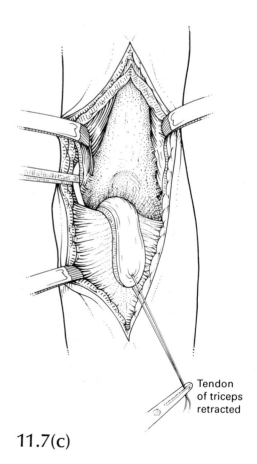

Tendon
of triceps
retracted

11.7(c)

distally across the olecranon and over the posterior border of the ulna extending 5 cm past the tip of the olecranon. The olecranon should be avoided by taking the incision just lateral to it (Figure 11.7(a)).

Approach

The skin, superficial and deep fascia are incised in line with the skin incision and are undercut as far as the medial and lateral humeral epicondyles. This exposes the triceps tendon (Figure 11.8(a)).

For further exposure of the distal humerus and elbow joint, the ulnar nerve is identified along the medial triceps margin and is dissected free enough to allow it to be encircled and protected by a moist tape. The olecranon is exposed by subperiosteal elevation of the flexor carpi ulnaris medially and of the anconeus laterally.

The distal humerus and elbow joint are then exposed either by splitting the triceps tendon (Figure 11.8(a)), or by olecranon osteotomy (Figure 11.8(b),(c)).

If olecranon osteotomy is chosen for exposure, the olecranon is then divided either intra-articularly (Figure 11.8(ci),(cii)) or extra-articularly (Figure 11.8(civ)). Prior to osteotomy, drilling for K-wires for tension band fixation (Figure 11.8(ciii)), or drilling and tapping for cancellous screw fixation (Figure 11.8(cv),(d)) will facilitate later olecranon fixation (Figure 11.8(c),(d)). An extra-articular cut spares the trochlear notch from damage but is more susceptible to non-union and limits the view of the trochlea, while an intra-articular osteotomy breaches the articular surface of the trochlear notch. If an extra-articular osteotomy is performed it is done obliquely in a single plane with either a saw, or preferably a thin, sharp osteotome, the subchondral bone being finally fractured rather than cut. If intra-articular osteotomy is done it may be transverse or 'chevronned'. Intra-articular osteotomy must be done by sharp, thin osteotome to avoid loss of bone. The proximal fragment of the osteotomized olecranon is then taken with the distal triceps tendon, which is incised laterally to separate it from the anconeus and medially, while gradually dissecting it, distal to proximal, from the posterior surface of the humerus (Figure 11.8(d)). Again, it is important to emphasize that care should be taken not to injure the ulnar nerve.

During closure of this incision, it is essential to restore the osteotomized olecranon process anatomically. It may be possible to preserve the position of the ulnar nerve in the cubital groove, provided it does not sublux during elbow motion. If it is does sublux during elbow motion, anterior transposition of the nerve should be considered. It is vitally important to document this anterior transposition in the operative record for future reference in the event of further surgery (such as implant removal) being necessary.

Indications

This is the approach of choice for restoration of comminuted intra-articular fractures of the distal humerus. Delayed or non-unions also can be treated through

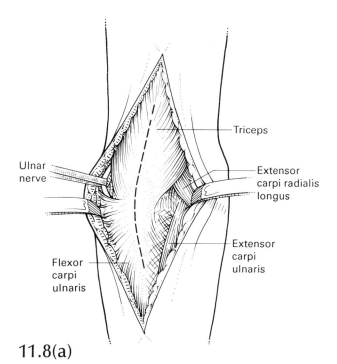

11.8(a)

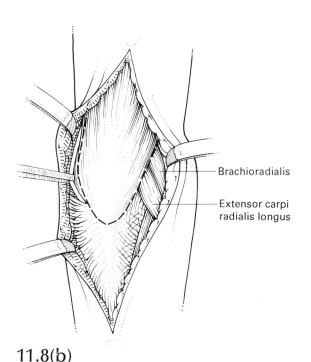

11.8(b)

this incision. It is suitable for arthrodesis and certain arthroplastic procedures of the elbow. It can be used for synovectomy, for resection of the olecranon and for the resection of heterotopic bone. This approach may be used without olecranon osteotomy for correction of snapping triceps, to harvest the triceps for tendon transfer, in certain methods of reconstructing a chronically dislocating elbow joint, in attaching a tendon transfer to enhance triceps strength or to repair a triceps avulsion.

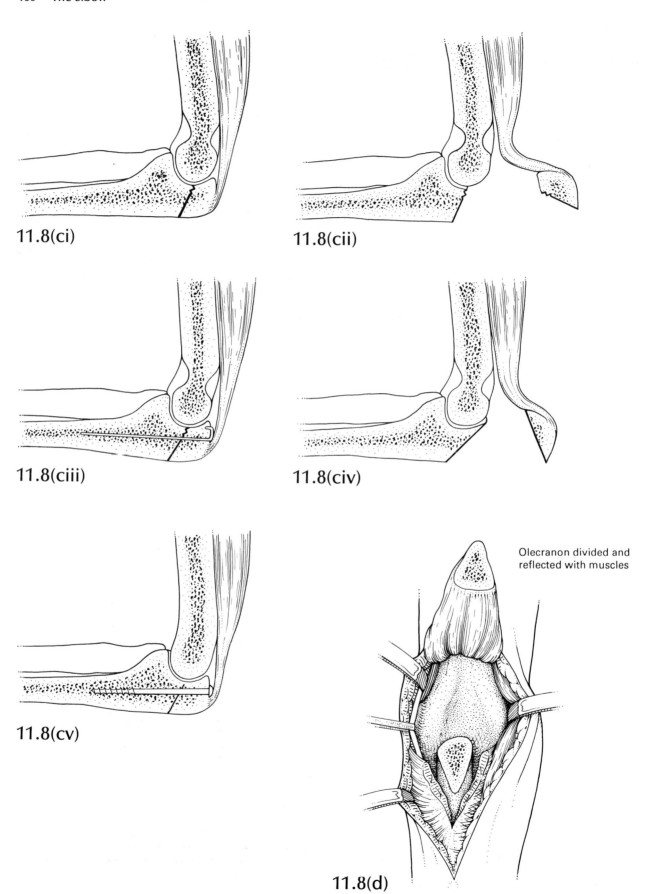

11.8(ci)

11.8(cii)

11.8(ciii)

11.8(civ)

11.8(cv)

Olecranon divided and
reflected with muscles

11.8(d)

Posterior approach – transolecranon 'U' (MacAusland)

Access

This approach provides access to the distal humerus including its articular surface.

Position

The patient may be positioned as for the other posterior approaches.

Incision

The incision is started at the lateral epicondyle of the humerus and extends distally and medially to cross the ulna 5 cm distal to the tip of the olecranon and is then continued proximally and medially to the medial humeral epicondyle. Proximal extensions of both sides of this 'U' incision may be taken as far proximally as necessary for the exposure desired (Figure 11.9).

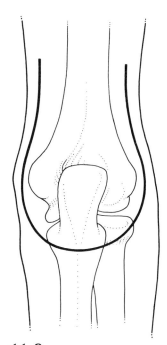

11.9

Approach

The distal portion of the flap is retracted proximally and the olecranon is exposed. The ulnar nerve is identified, exposed and protected with a moist tape. The olecranon is then osteotomized as already discussed. The proximal osteotomized olecranon is then taken with the skin,

subcutaneous tissue and triceps tendon and muscle as a single flap. If the skin and subcutaneous tissue are elevated as a flap separate from the triceps, skin necrosis can occur with this U-shaped incision. As this single myocutaneous flap is developed, dissection is carried laterally to separate it from the anconeus, medially from the ulnar nerve and extraperiosteally from distal to proximal along the posterior surface of the humerus. During closure it is essential to restore the osteotomized olecranon process anatomically. It may be possible to preserve the position of the ulnar nerve in the cubital groove, provided it does not sublux during elbow motion. If it does sublux during elbow motion, anterior transposition of the nerve should be considered, but it should be remembered that this procedure can be difficult to perform adequately through this incision. It is vitally important to document the anterior transposition in the operative record for future reference in the event of further surgery (such as implant removal) being necessary.

Indications

This approach can be used for open reduction and internal fixation of comminuted intra-articular distal humeral fractures, as well as for delayed or non-unions. It may also be used for certain arthroplastic procedures, for resection of the olecranon, arthrotomy and removal of loose bodies and synovectomy. The theoretical advantage of this incision over a straight incision is the wider exposure, although this is arguable.

Lateral approach

Access

This incision gives access to the lateral humeral epicondyle, capitellum, anterior and posterior compartments of the elbow, radial head, and the radial collateral and annular ligaments.

Position

The patient is supine on the operating table. The arm rests on an adjacent well-padded table, with the arm abducted and internally rotated. The elbow is flexed and its lateral aspect faces the surgeon.

Incision

The incision starts on the lateral supracondylar ridge 5 cm proximal to the elbow joint. It is extended distally on the lateral surface of the proximal forearm just posterior to the radial head for a distance of 5 cm from the elbow joint (Figure 11.10(a)).

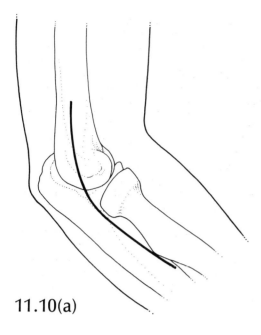

11.10(a)

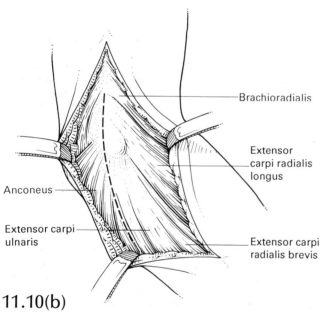

Brachioradialis

Extensor
carpi radialis
longus

Anconeus

Extensor carpi
ulnaris

Extensor carpi
radialis brevis

11.10(b)

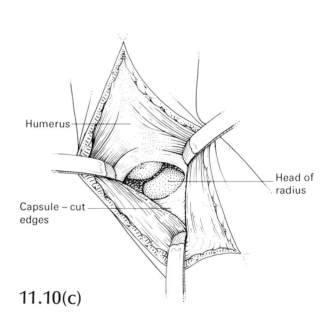

Humerus

Capsule – cut
edges

Head of
radius

11.10(c)

Approach

The skin and subcutaneous tissue are mobilized adequately for wide retraction and exposure. The deep fascia is
incised in line with the incision (Figure 11.10(b)). The
interval between the triceps muscle posteriorly and the
brachioradialis and extensor carpi radialis longus muscles
anteriorly is developed subperiosteally to expose the
lateral humeral epicondyle, lateral joint capsule and radial
collateral ligament. Take care to avoid injuring the deep
posterior interosseous motor branch of the radial nerve
which lies close to the anterior articular capsule over the
head of the radius. The dissection is then continued

distally between the extensor carpi ulnaris and the
anconeus. The supinator lies deep to and between the
anconeus and the extensor carpi ulnaris. The joint capsule
(radial collateral ligament) is incised longitudinally over
the lateral aspect of the head of the radius to expose the
articular surface of the head of the radius and the lower
end of the lateral humeral epicondyle and the capitellum
(Figure 11.10(c)). Further subperiosteal reflection of the
brachioradialis, extensor carpi radialis longus and common extensor origins anteriorly and the triceps posteriorly
from the lateral epicondylar ridge and detachment of the
anconeus from the ulna distally, will improve joint
exposure.

Indications

This exposure is suitable for surgery of fractures of the lateral humeral epicondyle, the capitellum and the head and neck of the radius. It is excellent for correcting radial head dislocation that is irreducible by closed methods. Arthrotomy can be performed for joint sepsis, removal of loose bodies or foreign bodies, the treatment of adjacent bone infection, tumour resection, synovectomy, radial head surgery, anterolateral joint capsulectomy for flexion contracture and the removal of heterotopic bone. Exploration of lateral epicondylitis (tennis elbow) and repair or partial excision of the annular ligament may be done through this approach. The chronically unstable elbow can be reconstructed using this lateral route.

Osteotomy of the lateral epicondyle with forward retraction of the attached muscle origins can greatly enhance the exposure of the radial head. The epicondyle is fixed back into position at the end of the procedure using a lag screw.

Posterolateral approach (Kocher)

Access

This incision gives access to the lateral humeral epicondyle, capitellum, anterior and posterior compartments of the elbow, radial head, radial collateral ligament and annular ligament.

Position

The patient is placed as for the preceding lateral approach (see p. 167).

Incision

The incision begins over the lateral aspect of the distal third of the humerus 5 cm above the elbow. It extends downward over the lateral epicondylar ridge across the elbow joint at the level of the radial head: 5 cm distally it is curved medially and posteriorly to end at the posterior subcutaneous margin of the ulna (Figure 11.11(a)).

Approach

The skin and cutaneous tissue are mobilized adequately for wide retraction and exposure. The deep fascia is incised in line with the incision (Figure 11.11(b)). The interval between the triceps muscle posteriorly and the brachioradialis and extensor carpi radialis longus muscles anteriorly is developed to expose the lateral humeral epicondyle, the lateral joint capsule and the radial collateral ligament. The dissection is continued distally as the fibres of the anconeus and the extensor carpi ulnaris are separated (Figure 11.11(c)). The supinator lies deep to

and between the anconeus and the extensor carpi ulnaris. The joint capsule (radial collateral ligament) is incised longitudinally to gain access to the joint (Figure 11.11(c),(d)). Subperiosteal reflection of the brachioradialis, extensor carpi radialis longus, common extensor origin and anterior capsule, the triceps and posterior capsule posteriorly from the humerus and of the anconeus from the ulna distally will complete the exposure of the elbow joint and even allow its operative lateral dislocation for still wider exposure (Figure 11.11(e)). To accomplish this the supinator is reflected downward and anteriorly by subperiosteal dissection from the ulna and the olecranon process is freed by subperiosteal dissection. The annular ligament may be divided to expose the radial neck. During this procedure the radial nerve is protected by the brachioradialis lateral to it, the deep posterior interosseous branch is protected within the two heads of the supinator and the nerve to the anconeus is protected within the triceps and anconeus substance. If the dissection is carried towards the medial humeral epicondyle, the ulnar nerve must be identified and protected.

Indications

This approach can be used for each of the procedures listed under the lateral approach. The advantage of this approach is a wider exposure of the elbow joint. It therefore has an advantage in performing synovectomy and searching for loose or foreign bodies and can, in addition, be used for certain arthroplastic procedures or arthrodesis.

Anterior approach (Pheasant)

Access

This approach affords access to the contents of the antecubital fossa and to the brachialis insertion, the coronoid process of the ulna, the anterior capsule of the elbow and, in some instances, to structures immediately adjacent to the antecubital fossa.

Position

The patient is supine on the operating table, with the contralateral shoulder and hip bolstered slightly, turning the patient towards the involved extremity. The arm is extended on an adjacent well-padded side-table, with the shoulder abducted and externally rotated.

Incision

The incision starts 5 cm above the elbow adjacent to the medial edge of the biceps muscle, extends distally between the medial biceps and the lateral border of the

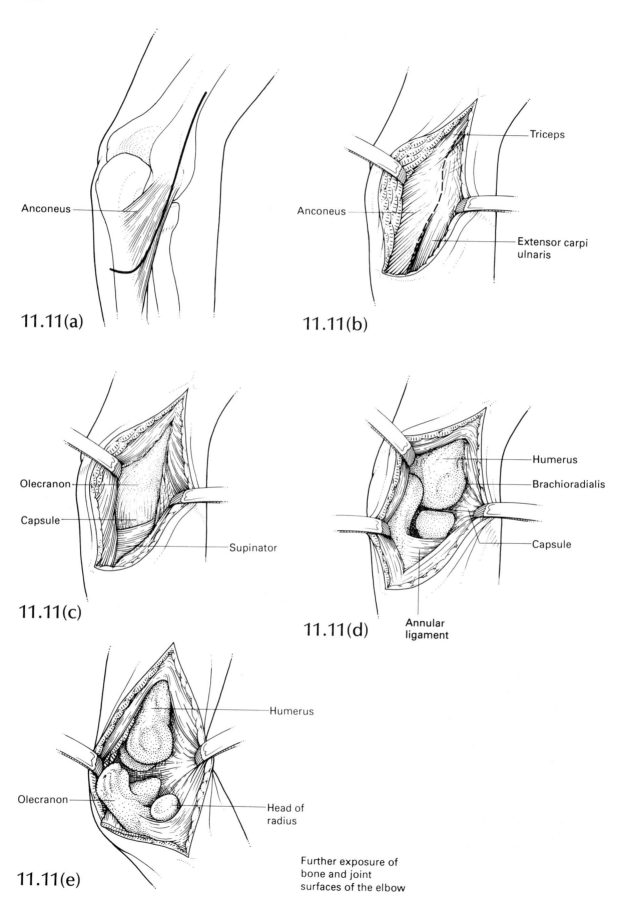

11.11(a)

Anconeus

11.11(b)

Triceps

Anconeus

Extensor carpi
ulnaris

11.11(c)

Olecranon

Capsule

Supinator

11.11(d)

Humerus

Brachioradialis

Capsule

Annular
ligament

11.11(e)

Olecranon

Humerus

Head of
radius

Further exposure of
bone and joint
surfaces of the elbow

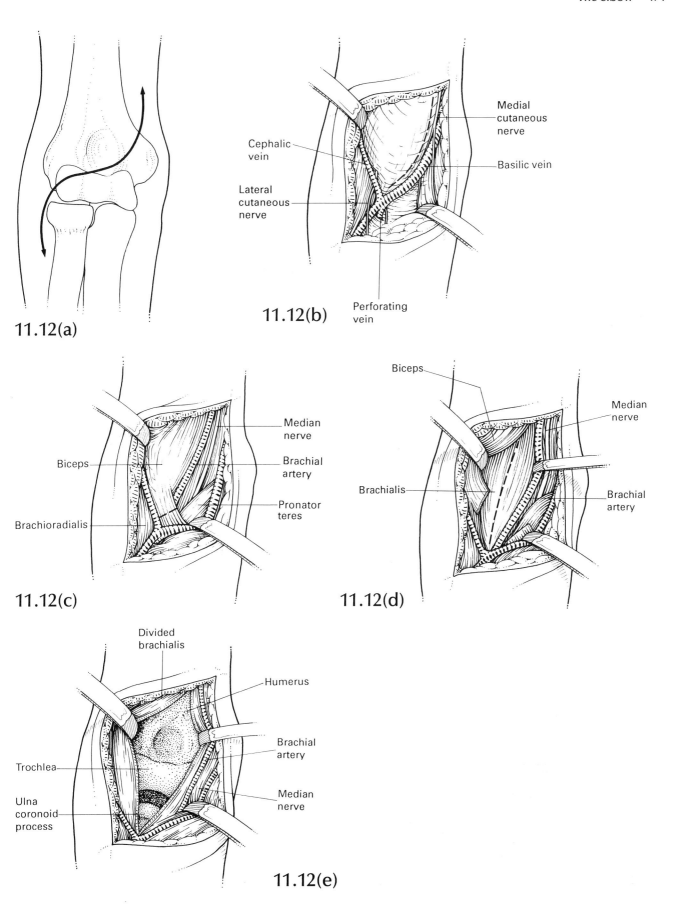

11.12(a)

11.12(b)

Cephalic vein

Lateral cutaneous nerve

Medial cutaneous nerve

Basilic vein

Perforating vein

11.12(c)

Biceps

Brachioradialis

Median nerve

Brachial artery

Pronator teres

11.12(d)

Biceps

Brachialis

Median nerve

Brachial artery

11.12(e)

Divided brachialis

Humerus

Brachial artery

Median nerve

Trochlea

Ulna coronoid process

pronator teres to the flexor crease of the elbow which it then crosses obliquely and continues distally 5 cm from the elbow joint along the medial border of the brachio-radialis (Figure 11.12(a)). Straight-line incisions across the flexor surfaces of joints must be avoided because they give rise to flexion contractures. This incision can be extensile proximally with a medial incision of the arm and distally with the anterior radial approach to the forearm.

Approach

Although it may be necessary to ligate the median antecubital vein and other small veins while extending this incision through the superficial fascia, the cephalic and basilic veins should be preserved (Figure 11.12(b)). The lateral antebrachial cutaneous nerve emerging from the lateral side of the distal biceps tendon must also be spared. The deep fascia and lacertus fibrosus are incised in line with the incision (Figure 11.12(b),(c)). This exposes the contents of the antecubital fossa, from medial to lateral: the median nerve, the brachial artery and the biceps tendon (MAT). The insertion of the brachialis may be exposed by mobilizing the brachial artery and median nerve medially and the biceps tendon laterally (Figure 11.12(d)). The anterior capsule of the elbow and subsequently the anterior portion of the distal humerus and the coronoid process may be exposed by first mobilizing or splitting the brachialis and then by incising and mobilizing the anterior joint capsule (Figure 11.12(e)). The branches from the median nerve to the pronator teres must be protected.

Indications

This approach may be used for repair of injuries to the biceps tendon and for biceps tendon transfers. It is a particularly useful approach for immediate or early repair of unstable fracture-dislocations of the elbow associated with fractures of the coronoid process. It can be used to reconstruct the elbow in cases of chronic instability and to relieve flexion contracture by biceps tendon lengthening, brachialis lengthening and anterior capsulotomy. Loose bodies in the anterior compartment of the elbow may be removed through this approach. This incision exposes the brachial artery and median nerve in the region of the elbow. The brachial artery may be disengaged if entrapped, repaired, controlled for embolectomy or reconstructed. The median nerve in this region may be decompressed, released from entrapment, repaired or reconstructed.

Medial approach (Molesworth, Campbell, Learmonth)

Access

This incision gives access to the ulnar nerve at the elbow, the medial humeral epicondyle and the medial elbow joint including the trochlea and the trochlear notch of the ulna.

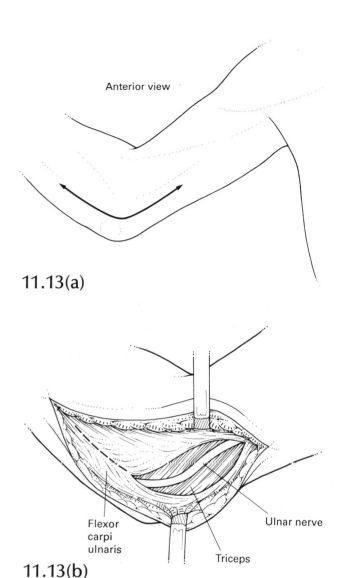

Anterior view

11.13(a)

Flexor carpi ulnaris

Ulnar nerve

Triceps

11.13(b)

Position

The patient is positioned supine and rolled slightly towards the involved upper extremity by padding under the contralateral shoulder and hip. The involved upper extremity is placed on a well-padded side-table, with the shoulder abducted and externally rotated and the elbow joint flexed.

Incision

An incision is made from 5 cm above the elbow joint to 5 cm below the elbow joint, centred over the medial supracondylar ridge and the medial epicondyle (Figure 11.13(a)). When extending the incision through the subcutaneous tissue, injury to the posterior branch of the medial antebrachial cutaneous nerve should be avoided (Figure 11.1(a),(b)). The incision can be centred 1.5 cm anterior or posterior to the medial humeral epicondyle when the ulnar nerve is being specifically sought for

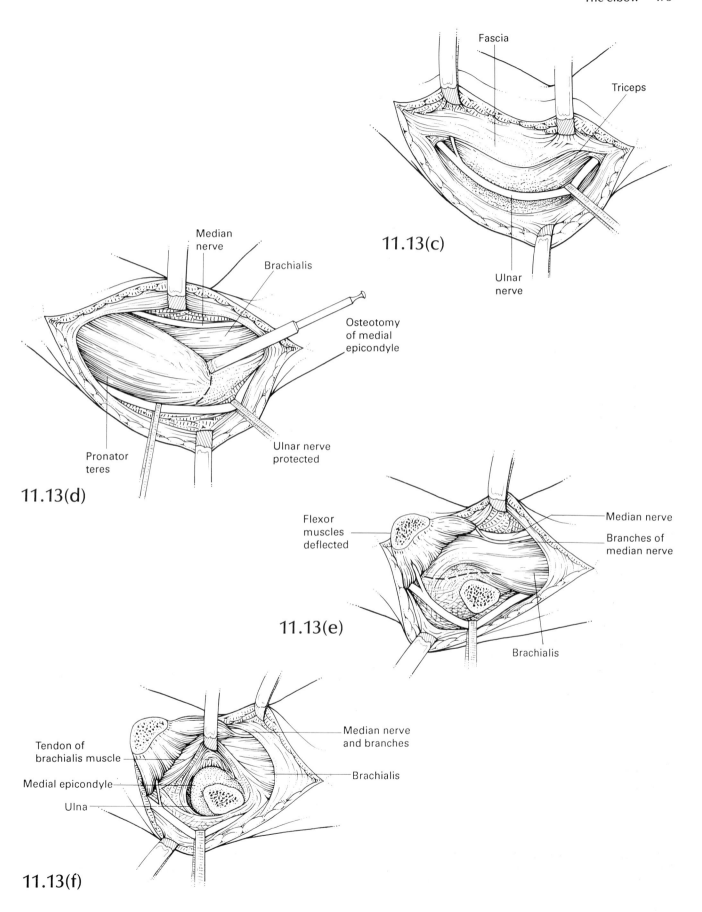

11.13(c)

Fascia

Triceps

Ulnar nerve

Median nerve

Brachialis

Osteotomy of medial epicondyle

Ulnar nerve protected

Pronator teres

11.13(d)

Flexor muscles deflected

Median nerve

Branches of median nerve

Brachialis

11.13(e)

Tendon of brachialis muscle

Medial epicondyle

Ulna

Median nerve and branches

Brachialis

11.13(f)

repair, decompression, grafting or anterior transposition, so as to avoid subsequent conflict between the scar and the bony prominence of the medial epicondyle. The incision and subsequent approach should be extended proximally and distally to release the ulnar nerve adequately when transposition is planned.

Approach

The ulnar nerve should be identified proximally in relation to the triceps, in its groove posterior to the medial epicondyle and distally in relation to its entry between the two heads of the flexor carpi ulnaris (Figure 11.13(b),(c)). When the nerve is entrapped or is being transposed, adequate decompression must be completed of the medial intermuscular septum proximally and of the epimysium and fascia of the flexor carpi ulnaris distally. The ulnar nerve should only be retracted by a moist tape. The first branch of the ulnar nerve is to the elbow joint and can be severed with impunity. The second branch is to the flexor carpi ulnaris and must be protected. The two can be distinguished anatomically and confirmed with a nerve stimulator.

The medial humeral epicondyle may be osteotomized and taken distally with the flexor pronator origin as far as the coronoid process (Figure 11.13(d),(e)). Branches of the median nerve enter the lateral border of the flexor pronator origin and must be respected. The median nerve lies on the brachialis just lateral to the pronator teres. The amount of exposure necessary dictates the extent of the dissection. The capsule is incised longitudinally and reflected anteriorly and posteriorly (Figure 11.13(e),(f)). For wider exposure of the elbow, the periosteum can be stripped with the capsule. The forearm can be abducted to wedge open the elbow joint, with the lateral capsule and radial collateral ligament complex acting as a hinge. In order to avoid osteotomy of the medial humeral epicondyle, a slightly posterior approach may be taken and the flexor pronator origin may be taken anteriorly with the ulnar nerve using subperiosteal dissection but leaving sufficient proximal attachment of the flexor pronator origin so that it may be reconstituted by suture at the conclusion of the procedure.

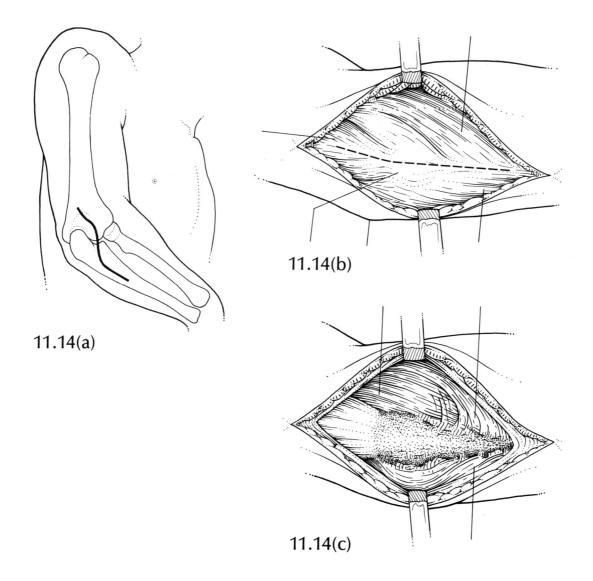

11.14(a)

11.14(b)

11.14(c)

Indications

This approach is used to repair displaced medial epicondylar fractures. It is used for decompression, transposition, repair or reconstruction of the ulnar nerve. In addition, it is used for certain arthroplasties, certain reconstructive procedures for chronic elbow instability and to remove heterotopic bone. It is also used in some instances to approach fractures of the coronoid process. It may be used alone or in conjunction with a lateral elbow incision for drainage of the elbow joint, removal of loose or foreign bodies, synovectomy and for release of the anteromedial joint capsule for flexion contracture. This incision may be used with an additional anterior incision to free the median nerve when it is entrapped between the medial humeral epicondyle and the trochlear notch in instances of posterior elbow dislocation.

Posterior approach – olecranon and proximal ulna

Access

This incision provides access to the olecranon process and proximal ulna.

Position

The patient is supine. The shoulder is adducted and the elbow flexed across the torso. The forearm is supinated.

Incision

The incision begins at the mid-line just above the tip of the olecranon and extends over the subcutaneous margin of the proximal ulna curving laterally to avoid crossing the bony prominence (Figure 11.14(a)).

Approach

The incision is carried through subcutaneous fat and then through the deep fascia in the mid-line of the ulna (Figure 11.14(b)). The periosteum is incised in the mid-line with the incision reflecting the extensor carpi ulnaris medially and the anconeus and supinator laterally by subperiosteal dissection: the ulnar nerve within the flexor carpi ulnaris muscle in the proximal forearm is thereby protected. More proximally, the ulnar nerve lies medial to the olecranon coming from the cubital groove of the medial humeral epicondyle. Identification and sufficient exposure are necessary to ensure its protection if the dissection is carried proximally (Figure 11.14(c)). The posterior capsule of the elbow joint may be exposed by this approach.

Indications

This incision may be used for the repair of olecranon and proximal ulnar fractures and for the excision of the olecranon.

References

Campbell, R. E. (1932) Incision for exposure of the elbow joint. *Am. J. Surg.*, **15**, 65
Learmonth, J. R. (1942) A technique for transplanting the ulnar nerve. *Surg. Gynecol. Obstet.*, **75**, 792
MacAusland Jr, W. R. and Wyman Jr, E. T. (1975) Fractures of the adult elbow. In *American Academy of Orthopedic Surgeons: Instructional Course Lectures*, vol. 24, C. V. Mosby, St Louis, p. 169
Molesworth, W. H. L. (1930) Operation for complete exposure of the elbow joint. *Br. J. Surg.*, **18**, 303
Van Gorder, G. W. (1932) Surgical approach in old posterior dislocation of the elbow. *J. Bone Joint Surg.*, **14A**, 127
Van Gorder, G. W. (1940) Surgical approach in supracondylar 'T' fractures of the humerus requiring open reduction. *J. Bone Joint Surg.*, **22**, 278

Further reading

Spinner, M. and Kaplan, E. B. (1970) The quadrate ligament of the elbow: its relationship to the stability of the proximal radioulnar joint. *Acta Orthop. Scand.*, **41**, 632

Chapter 12

The forearm

A. E. Freeland and J. L. Hughes

RELEVANT ANATOMY

Superficial cutaneous nerves

The superficial cutaneous nerves in the forearm may develop painful neuromas if they are divided, particularly the posterior branch of the medial antebrachial cutaneous nerve in the proximal forearm and the dorsal sensory branch of the radial nerve in the distal forearm. Incisions and approaches should therefore be planned to spare these nerves whenever possible. Conversely, the lateral antebrachial cutaneous nerve is an excellent donor for interfascicular nerve grafts, especially of the digital nerves, and complications from harvesting this nerve are rare.

LATERAL ANTEBRACHIAL CUTANEOUS NERVE (Figure 12.1)

The lateral antebrachial cutaneous nerve is a continuation of the musculocutaneous nerve. It surfaces from behind the biceps, just lateral to the biceps tendon, and pierces the deep fascia at the level of the elbow to lie behind and between the cephalic and accessory cephalic veins. It then divides into anterior and posterior branches. The anterior branch continues distally along the radial half of the anterior surface of the forearm supplying the skin in this area. It is superficial to the radial artery at the wrist and terminates by dividing with the radial artery, some filaments supplying the proximal thenar eminence and

others going with the deep branch to the dorsal surface of the carpus. The posterior branch courses on the radial side of the forearm to the wrist supplying the overlying skin and the skin on the very radial side of the back of the forearm.

MEDIAL ANTEBRACHIAL CUTANEOUS NERVE (Figure 12.1)

The main trunk of the medial antebrachial cutaneous nerve leaves the medial side of the brachial artery and pierces the deep fascia at mid-arm with the basilic vein. It then divides into anterior and posterior branches. The anterior branch continues adjacent to the median vein on the ulnar side of the anterior forearm as far as the wrist, supplying overlying skin. The posterior branch parallels the medial side of the basilic vein running obliquely anterior to the medial humeral epicondyle and to the dorso-ulnar aspect of the forearm where it continues to the wrist, supplying overlying skin.

POSTERIOR ANTEBRACHIAL CUTANEOUS NERVE (Figure 12.1(b))

The posterior antebrachial cutaneous nerve is one of the lateral group of radial nerve branches. It pierces the lateral head of the triceps just before the radial nerve goes forwards through the lateral intermuscular septum. It then penetrates the brachial fascia to run posteriorly to the lateral humeral epicondyle and courses down the middle of the posterior forearm as far as the wrist, supplying the overlying skin between the posterior branches of the lateral and medial antebrachial cutaneous nerves.

176

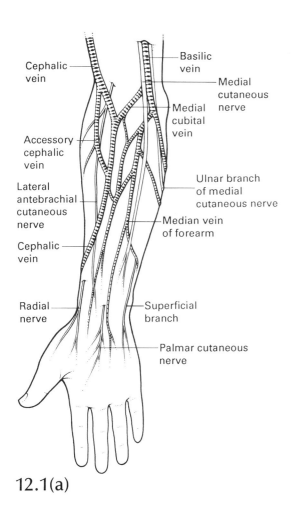

Cephalic vein

Basilic vein

Medial cutaneous nerve

Medial cubital vein

Accessory cephalic vein

Ulnar branch of medial cutaneous nerve

Lateral antebrachial cutaneous nerve

Median vein of forearm

Cephalic vein

Radial nerve

Superficial branch

Palmar cutaneous nerve

12.1(a)

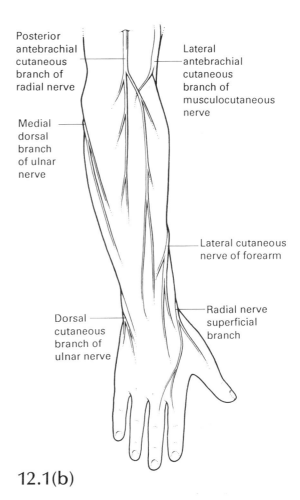

Posterior antebrachial cutaneous branch of radial nerve

Lateral antebrachial cutaneous branch of musculocutaneous nerve

Medial dorsal branch of ulnar nerve

Lateral cutaneous nerve of forearm

Dorsal cutaneous branch of ulnar nerve

Radial nerve superficial branch

12.1(b)

Deep nerves and vessels

MEDIAN NERVE (Figures 12.2–12.4)

The median nerve traverses the antecubital fossa anterior to the brachialis and medial to the brachial artery. It enters the forearm by coursing obliquely from medial to lateral over the ulnar artery and between the two heads of the pronator teres, the deep head separating it from the ulnar artery. It then runs distally just lateral to the ulnar artery and superficial to the flexor digitorum profundus. It runs between the two heads of the flexor digitorum superficialis and then deep to this muscle, being invested with its posterior fascia. In the distal forearm it surfaces from behind the superficial flexor, just to the lateral side of its tendons. It then proceeds anteriorly to lie consistently between the superficial flexor tendons to the index and middle fingers at the wrist, posterolateral to palmaris longus (PL to PL). It also lies just medial and posterior to the flexor carpi radialis tendon.

The branch or branches of the median nerve to the pronator teres are usually given off in the antecubital fossa, and are discussed in Chapter 11 on the elbow. The branches to the flexor carpi radialis, palmaris longus and flexor digitorum superficialis are given off sequentially

and proximal to the anterior interosseous nerve, except for one branch to the flexor digitorum superficialis to the index finger, which may be given off as much as 20 cm below the medial epicondyle and occasionally from the anterior interosseous nerve itself. Usually there is a single motor branch each to the flexor carpi radialis and the palmaris longus, but there are usually two or more branches to the flexor digitorum superficialis. There may also be branches of the median nerve to the radial part of the flexor digitorum profundus and to the flexor pollicis longus proximal to the anterior interosseous nerve.

The anterior interosseous nerve is the largest branch of the median nerve and arises about 5 cm distal to the medial epicondyle (Figures 12.3, 12.4). It runs obliquely from medial to lateral across the upper lateral portion of the flexor digitorum profundus. It then descends between this muscle and the flexor pollicis longus, on top of the interosseous membrane, with the anterior interosseous artery on its medial side. It gives off two or more branches both to the flexor digitorum profundus and the flexor pollicis longus. It consistently supplies at least the flexor digitorum profundus to the index finger. It terminates deep to the pronator quadratus by dividing to supply this muscle and to give branches to the anterior wrist capsule.

The palmar cutaneous nerve often arises from the anterior surface of the median nerve just above the wrist

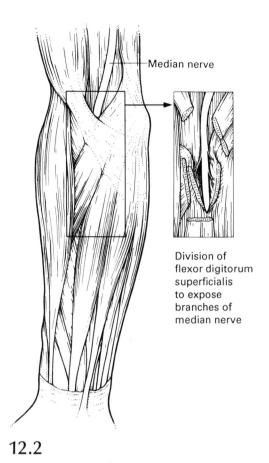

Division of
flexor digitorum
superficialis
to expose
branches of
median nerve

12.2

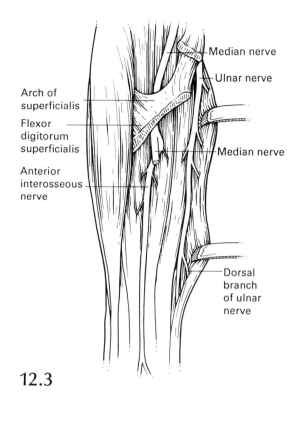

12.3

and pierces the deep fascia to become subcutaneous and
divide into radial and ulnar branches over the thenar
eminence while the median nerve enters the carpal tunnel
under the retinaculum and transverse carpal ligament
(Figure 12.1(a)).

ULNAR NERVE (Figures 12.3, 12.4)

The ulnar nerve enters the forearm between the humeral
and ulnar heads of the flexor carpi ulnaris, then lies deep
to this muscle, on top of the flexor digitorum profundus.
It runs straight down the forearm to the wrist and is joined
on its lateral side at the mid-forearm level by the ulnar
artery. The ulnar nerve and artery continue together to the
wrist, where they surface just lateral to the flexor carpi
ulnaris tendon and pass lateral to the pisiform bone.

The branches (usually two) of the ulnar nerve to the
flexor carpi ulnaris are given off in the elbow region
proximal to this muscle. The branch to the flexor
digitorum profundus is usually single and arises below, or
in concert with, the second branch to the flexor carpi
ulnaris, about 3 cm below the medial humeral epicondyle.
The branch from the ulnar nerve usually supplies the
medial half of the flexor digitorum profundus.

The ulnar nerve has two cutaneous branches that arise
distally in the forearm: the posterior ulnar cutaneous
branch arises about 7 cm proximal to the tip of the ulnar
styloid and the palmar cutaneous branch arises from the

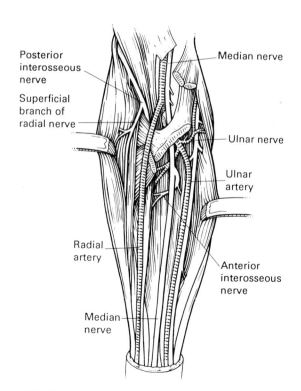

12.4

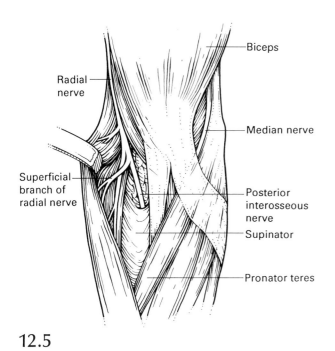

12.5

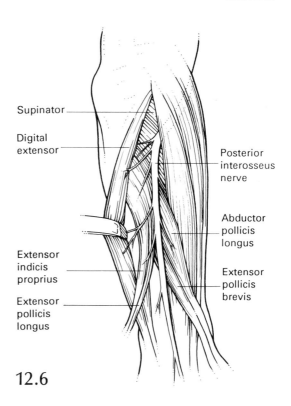

12.6

nerve in the mid or distal forearm. The posterior ulnar cutaneous branch becomes subcutaneous about 3 cm above the ulnar styloid, going dorsally between the ulna and the ulnar border of the flexor carpi ulnaris.

The palmar cutaneous branch runs subcutaneously with the ulnar artery to the skin of the palm.

RADIAL NERVE (Figures 12.4, 12.5)

At a level from 4 cm above to 4 cm below the tip of the lateral humeral condyle, the radial nerve divides into a deep motor branch, the posterior interosseous nerve, and a superficial sensory branch. The bifurcation is usually below the tip of the lateral humeral condyle. At this level, one, or sometimes two, branches are given off to the extensor carpi radialis brevis usually from the deep motor branch, less often from the superficial sensory branch and only rarely from the main trunk at or above the bifurcation.

The posterior interosseous nerve (Figures 12.4–12.6) is a purely motor nerve except for its distribution to the wrist joint where it terminates. It enters the upper edge of the superficial lamina of the supinator muscle through the arcade of Frohse. It enters the forearm between the two heads of the supinator, which it supplies with several branches both above and within the muscle. If the insertion of the deep head of the supinator parallels the nerve, the nerve may lie on the radius just below this insertion, where it is most likely to be injured by fracture or by the surgeon.

After the posterior interosseous nerve emerges from the lower margin of the supinator, it branches superficially to supply in turn the superficial group of extensor muscles of the forearm, the extensor digitorum communis, the extensor digiti minimi and the extensor carpi ulnaris (Figure 12.6) although the number and sequence of branches to the superficial extensor muscles can be quite variable. The abductor pollicis longus, extensor pollicis brevis, extensor pollicis longus and extensor indicis proprius are usually supplied by the posterior interosseous nerve in this order. The posterior interosseous nerve then continues across the superficial surface of the abductor pollicis longus, gives off one or more branches to the deep extensor muscles and then continues on the posterior surface of the interosseous membrane, deep to the extensor pollicis longus and extensor indicis proprius, to terminate in a gangliform enlargement at the back of the wrist.

The superficial branch of the radial nerve may give off a branch to the extensor carpi radialis brevis but is otherwise purely sensory (Figure 12.4). It runs distally beneath the brachioradialis, obliquely from anterior to posterior, to surface at the dorsal border of the brachioradialis tendon at the junction of the middle and distal thirds of the forearm (Figure 12.1(b)).

ULNAR ARTERY (Figures 12.4–12.7)

The ulnar artery enters the forearm beneath the pronator teres and then joins the median nerve, which lies lateral to it, between the two heads of the flexor digitorum superficialis. It continues distally and medially, emerging from behind the ulnar border of the flexor digitorum superficialis to lie under cover of the flexor carpi ulnaris, between this muscle and the flexor digitorum profundus. It is lateral and adjacent to the ulnar nerve and surfaces with it just lateral to the flexor carpi ulnaris tendon at the wrist. They pass lateral to the pisiform at the wrist and

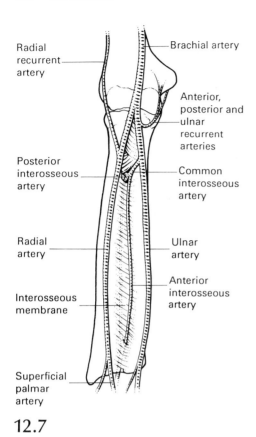

12.7

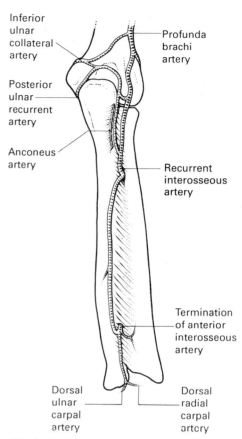

12.8

there the ulnar artery gives off palmar and dorsal carpal branches.

The ulnar artery gives off most of its named branches under cover of the flexor digitorum superficialis (Figures 12.4–12.7). The first branch of the ulnar artery, the ulnar recurrent artery, together with the interosseous recurrent artery, form important links in the collateral circulation around the elbow and are discussed in Chapter 11.

The common interosseous artery arises from the dorsolateral aspect of the ulnar artery about 2.5 cm from its origin (Figure 12.7). It passes posterior to the median nerve and divides immediately into the anterior and posterior interosseous arteries. The anterior interosseous artery courses distally on the anterior surface of the interosseous membrane, between the flexor digitorum profundus and the flexor pollicis longus, supplying both muscles. Proximally it gives off the median artery. It lies medial to the anterior interosseous nerve. The anterior interosseous artery gives rise to the nutrient arteries of both the radius and ulna and terminates by dividing into anterior and posterior branches at the superior border of the pronator quadratus muscle, the posterior branch passing dorsally through a gap in the distal part of the interosseous membrane.

The posterior interosseous artery passes dorsally between the radius and ulna, either above the oblique cord or between the oblique cord and the interosseous membrane, to emerge between the lower border of the supinator and the upper border of the abductor pollicis longus (Figures 12.7, 12.8). It sends branches to the superficial extensor muscles, gives off the recurrent

interosseous artery and then continues distally, with the posterior interosseous nerve, across the abductor pollicis longus. The posterior interosseous artery then leaves the posterior interosseous nerve, where the nerve passes deep to the extensor pollicis longus, and comes to lie on the posterior surface of the interosseous membrane. The posterior interosseous artery remains between the deep extensor muscles, supplying them and anastomosing with the posterior branch of the anterior interosseous artery at the distal portion of the interosseous membrane.

RADIAL ARTERY (Figures 12.4, 12.7)

The radial artery runs laterally and distally over the biceps tendon, the supinator and the insertion of pronator teres, coming to lie beneath the medial border of the brachioradialis belly. It continues medial to the superficial sensory branch of the radial nerve and lies anterior and lateral to the flexor digitorum superficialis. It then comes to lie anterior to the flexor pollicis longus and later the pronator quadratus. It is superficial to the deep antebrachial fascia, is extracompartmental and lies between the tendons of flexor carpi radialis and brachioradialis, where it is palpable at the wrist. Just proximal to the wrist, the radial artery divides into the superficial and deep branches. The superficial branch continues subcutaneously, over the muscles of the thenar eminence, to the superficial palmar arch, while the deep branch passes deep to the tendons of the first dorsal compartment, obliquely across the anatomical snuff box, to the angle between the thumb and index metacarpals.

The first branch of the radial artery, the radial recurrent artery, is an important contributor to the collateral circulation around the elbow (Figure 12.7). There are many unnamed muscular branches along its course.

Anterior (flexor) compartment of the forearm

The deep antebrachial fascia encircles the forearm and is continuous with the fascia of the arm above and the hand below. It is attached to the subcutaneous border of the ulna and it sends a septum to the radius dividing the anterior (flexor) and posterior (extensor) compartments of the forearm.

Proximally, the deep antebrachial fascia covers the flexor muscles and sends septa between them. These muscles take partial origin from the deep antebrachial fascia and these intervening septa. In the lower forearm, the deep antebrachial fascia divides into two layers. The thin superficial layer covers the flexor carpi radialis, palmaris longus and flexor carpi ulnaris, reinforced at the wrist with transverse fibres to form the volar carpal ligament. The thicker, deep layer lies between these three superficial wrist flexors and the digitial flexors. It, too, is strengthened at the wrist with transverse fibres to form the flexor retinaculum.

SUPERFICIAL MUSCLE GROUP (Figure 12.9)

The superficial muscles of the anterior forearm are four and include, from proximal to distal and from lateral to medial, pronator teres, flexor carpi radialis, palmaris longus and flexor carpi ulnaris.

The pronator teres originates from two heads – humeral and ulnar. The humeral head, larger and more superficial, arises from the common tendon of the flexor pronator origin, immediately above the medial humeral epicondyle. The much smaller ulnar head originates from the medial side of the coronoid process of the ulna, beneath the attachment of the flexor digitorum superficialis, to join the humeral head at an acute angle. They pass obliquely across the forearm to form a flat tendon that inserts in a rough area on the lateral surface of the middle third of the radius.

The flexor carpi radialis originates from the medial humeral epicondyle, via the common tendon of origin of the flexor pronator group. It lies medial to the pronator teres and lateral to the palmaris longus and ends in a long tendon that passes through a canal in the lateral part of the flexor retinaculum. It occupies a synovial sheath in a volar groove on the trapezium and inserts into the base of the second metacarpal, sending a slip to the base of the third metacarpal.

The palmaris longus arises from the common tendon of

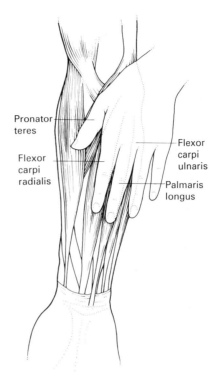

12.9

origin of the flexor pronator muscle group at the medial humeral epicondyle. It arborizes distally to insert into the palmar fascia.

The flexor carpi ulnaris is the most medial of the superficial flexor muscle group. It arises by two heads, humeral and ulnar, connected by a tendinous arch. The small humeral head arises from the common flexor pronator tendinous origin at the medial humeral epicondyle. The large ulnar head arises from the medial olecranon and the upper two-thirds of the posterior border of the ulna. The ulnar nerve and posterior recurrent ulnar artery pass between these two heads. It inserts into the pisiform bone and indirectly into the volar hamate and fifth metacarpal via the piso-hamate and piso-metacarpal ligaments. It is supplied by the ulnar nerve.

INTERMEDIATE FLEXOR MUSCLE GROUP

The flexor digitorum superficialis (Figures 12.10, 12.11) has two heads, humero-ulnar and radial. The humero-ulnar head arises from the common tendon at the medial humeral epicondyle, from the anterior band of the ulnar collateral ligament of the elbow and from the medial side of the coronoid process of the ulna, above the origin of the pronator teres. The radial head arises from the anterior border of the radius between the radial tuberosity and the pronator teres insertion. The median nerve and ulnar artery pass between and deep to these two heads.

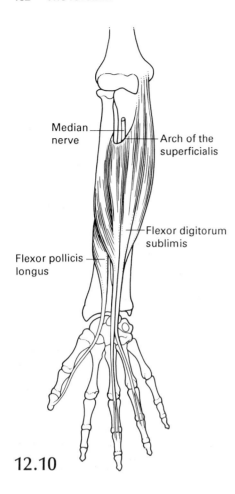

12.10

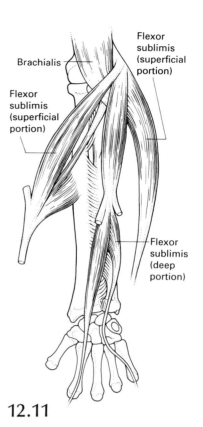

12.11

The muscle forms two strata, a superficial one for the middle and ring fingers and a deep one for the index and little fingers. This muscle is posterior to all of the superficial wrist flexors, and to the radial artery and nerve. It lies anterior to flexor digitorum profundus, the proximal ulnar artery, the median nerve and flexor pollicis longus.

DEEP ANTERIOR MUSCLE GROUP (Figure 12.12)

The flexor digitorum profundus arises from the proximal three-quarters of the anterior surface of the ulna between the brachialis insertion and the pronator quadratus origin, deep to the flexor digitorum superficialis, from a depression on the coronoid process and from the ulnar half of the front of the interosseous membrane. There are four tendons that insert into the bases of the distal phalanges of their respective digits. The lateral part of the muscle is supplied by the anterior interosseous branch of the median nerve and the medial half by the ulnar nerve.

The flexor pollicis longus is lateral to the flexor digitorum profundus. It arises from the grooved anterior radius, from the tuberosity to the insertion of the pronator quadratus and from the radial side of the adjacent interosseous membrane. The tendon passes through the carpal tunnel to insert on the base of the distal phalanx of the thumb. The flexor pollicis longus is supplied by the anterior interosseous branch of the median nerve.

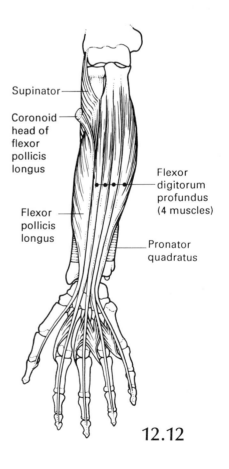

12.12

The pronator quadratus arises from the oblique ridge on the distal quarter of the anterior ulna and inserts into the distal quarter of the anterior surface of the radius. It is innervated by the anterior interosseous branch of the median nerve.

Posterior compartment of the forearm

The common fascial cylindrical sheath which envelopes the forearm is separated into anterior and posterior compartments by its attachment to the subcutaneous border of the ulna and by a fibrous septum to the lateral border of the radius. It covers the extensor muscles, along with septa which it drops between the muscles and thereby contributes to their origins. Distally, at the wrist, the posterior fascia thickens obliquely to form the compartmentalized extensor retinaculum. The posterior compartment of the forearm contains three groups of muscles, the 'mobile wad' of three muscles, the superficial group and the deep group.

'MOBILE WAD OF THREE' (Figure 12.13)

The brachioradialis and the extensor carpi radialis longus and brevis constitute the 'mobile wad of three' (Henry, 1927). These muscles may be regarded as a single

anatomical unit, which may be fully moved between the thumb and forefinger, and approaches to the forearm are made to either side of them.

The brachioradialis arises from the upper two-thirds of the lateral humeral supracondylar ridge and from the anterior aspect of the lateral intermuscular septum. It is the most superficial muscle of the radial forearm and forms the lateral border of the antecubital fossa. The radial nerve, radial recurrent artery and radial collateral artery are found between it and the brachialis. It forms a broad, flat tendon that inserts into the lateral aspect of the radial styloid process, where it is crossed by the tendons of the first dorsal compartment (abductor pollicis longus and extensor pollicis brevis). The radial artery parallels its medial side. It is supplied by the radial nerve.

The extensor carpi radialis longus arises from the lower third of the lateral humeral supracondylar ridge and the adjacent anterior surface of the lateral intermuscular septum of the arm. Its tendon runs deep to the abductor pollicis longus and extensor pollicis brevis on to the dorsal surface of the radial styloid through the second dorsal compartment of the wrist, with the extensor carpi radialis brevis tendon ulnar to it, and inserts on the dorsal base of the second metacarpal. It is supplied by the radial nerve.

The extensor carpi radialis brevis arises from the common extensor tendon of origin on the lateral humeral epicondyle and from the lateral collateral ligament of the elbow. It follows a course adjacent and medial to the extensor carpi radialis longus, through the second dorsal wrist compartment, to insert on the base of the third metacarpal. At the radius it is separated from the extensor carpi radialis longus by a ridge proximal to Lister's tubercle. This muscle is innervated usually from the posterior interosseous branch of the radial nerve.

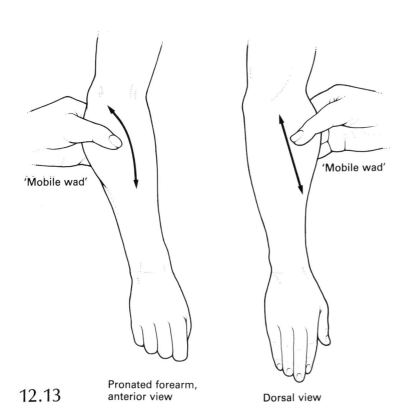

12.13

Pronated forearm,
anterior view

Dorsal view

SUPERFICIAL MUSCLE GROUP (Figure 12.14)

The extensor digitorum communis arises deep to the extensor carpi radialis brevis, from the common tendon on the lateral humeral condyle, and divides into four tendons which pass through the fourth dorsal compartment with the extensor indicis proprius. The extensor indicis proprius tendon is medial to the extensor digitorum communis tendon to the index finger. Each tendon of the extensor digitorum inserts into the dorsal digital expansion of its respective finger. The posterior interosseous nerve innervates this muscle through one or more of its superficial branches.

The extensor digiti quinti minimi arises from the common extensor origin on the lateral humeral epicondyle, distal to the extensor digitorum communis. Its tendon runs through the fifth dorsal wrist compartment, over the inferior radio-ulnar joint and then usually divides into two tendinous slips. Like the extensor indicis proprius, its tendon lies medial to its companion, the extensor digitorum communis tendon to the fifth finger. It is innervated by one or more superficial branches of the posterior interosseous nerve.

The extensor carpi ulnaris originates distal to the extensor digiti quinti minimi, from the common tendon on the lateral humeral epicondyle and from the posterior border of the ulna. It ends in a tendon that is alone in the sixth dorsal wrist compartment in a groove between the head and styloid process of the ulna. It inserts onto a tubercle on the medial side of the base of the fifth metacarpal and is supplied by superficial branches of the posterior interosseous nerve.

DEEP EXTENSOR MUSCLE GROUP (Figure 12.15)

The supinator arises by a superficial head via tendinous fibres and by a deep head through muscular fibres from the lateral humeral epicondyle, the lateral collateral ligament of the elbow, the annular ligament and the proximal supinator crest of the ulna. The supinator encircles the upper third of the radius attaching to its lateral surface and it contains the posterior interosseous nerve, which innervates it between its two heads. It supinates the forearm alone when the elbow is flexed and when motion is slow; it acts in concert with the biceps when the elbow is flexed and when motion faster. It acts alone at all speeds when the elbow is extended.

The abductor pollicis longus arises from the postero-lateral shaft of the ulna below the anconeus, from the posterior interosseous membrane and the posterior border of the middle third of the radius below the supinator insertion. The muscle and tendon pass obliquely, distally and laterally, just lateral to the tendon of the extensor pollicis brevis, with which it passes over the radial wrist extensors into the first dorsal wrist compartment, to split into two or more tendons which insert onto the base of the thumb metacarpal and the trapezium. This muscle is innervated by the posterior interosseous nerve and it radially abducts the thumb at the first carpometacarpal joint.

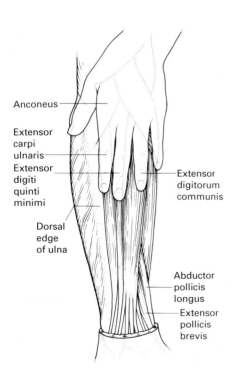

12.14   Dorsal aspect of forearm

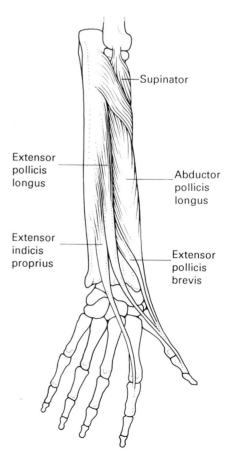

12.15

The extensor pollicis brevis arises from the posterior interosseous membrane and posterior surface of the radius distal to the abductor pollicis longus. It courses medial to this same companion through the first dorsal wrist compartment to attach to the base of the proximal phalanx of the thumb, just lateral to the extensor pollicis longus. It is innervated by the posterior interosseous nerve.

The extensor pollicis longus arises from the posterior interosseous membrane and the posterior surface of the radial shaft, distal to the extensor pollicis brevis. Its tendon passes alone through the third dorsal wrist compartment, medial to Lister's tubercle, in an oblique groove on the back of the distal radius, and then crosses superficial to the tendons of the radial wrist extensors, attaching to the dorsal base of the distal phalanx of the thumb, where it is joined by the abductor and the adductor pollicis brevis aponeuroses. It is innervated by the posterior interosseous nerve. It extends the interphalangeal joint of the thumb and after completing this action it acts as an accessory to assist in metacarpophalangeal extension and finally radial abduction.

The extensor indicis proprius is below and parallel to its above precursors and arises from the posterior interosseous membrane and posterior surface of the ulna. Its tendon passes through the fourth dorsal wrist compartment and remains medially adjacent to the extensor digitorum to the index finger until it inserts into the dorsal hood of the index metacarpophalangeal joint which it aids in extension. It is the last muscle innervated from the radial nerve in the forearm via the deep division of the posterior interosseous nerve.

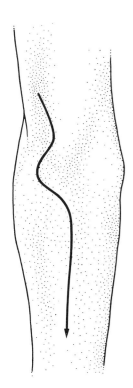

Anterior aspect   12.16

SURGICAL APPROACHES

- Proximal anterior for radius (Henry)
- Posterolateral (Speed and Boyd)
- Posterolateral (Thompson)
- Anterior distal (Henry)
- Combined posterior for radius and ulna

Radius – proximal anterior approach (Henry)

Access

This incision gives access to the distal radial nerve and to its deep posterior interosseous and superficial divisions, as well as to the proximal and middle thirds of the radial shaft.

Position

The patient is supine with the shoulder abducted and externally rotated. The upper extremity is placed on an adjacent arm table with the elbow extended and the forearm supinated.

Incision

This incision starts from the flexion crease of the elbow just lateral to the biceps tendon and runs parallel to the medial margin of the brachioradialis for a distance of 18 cm (Figure 12.16). It is extensile proximally, with either the anterior distal incision of the humerus (see p. 189) or the anterior (Pheasant) incision of the elbow (see p. 169) and distally with the anterior approach to the radius further down in the forearm.

Approach

The superficial and deep fascia are incised in line with the skin incision. The brachioradialis and 'mobile wad of three', are mobilized and retracted laterally, taking care to identify and protect the radial artery and the superficial branch of the radial nerve (Figure 12.17(a),(b)). The radial recurrent artery and veins are identified along with accessory branches and they are ligated and divided (Figure 12.17(b),(c)). This is an important step since a postoperative compartment syndrome can occur if they are cut and then allowed to retract without obtaining haemostasis. The pronator teres and flexor carpi radialis are retracted to the medial side. The brachioradialis and 'mobile wad' are retracted laterally to expose the supinator (Figure 12.18(a)). This manoeuvre may be facilitated by elbow flexion. The periosteum of the radius

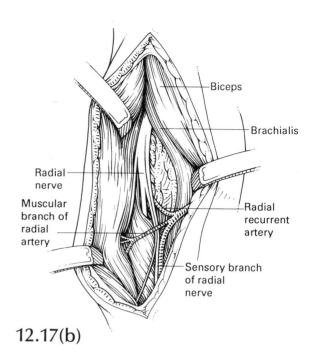

12.17(a)

Biceps

Brachialis

Brachioradialis

Radial artery

Pronator teres

12.17(b)

Biceps

Brachialis

Radial nerve

Muscular branch of radial artery

Radial recurrent artery

Sensory branch of radial nerve

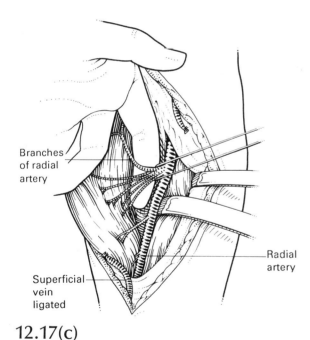

12.17(c)

Branches of radial artery

Radial artery

Superficial vein ligated

is incised between the supinator and the adjacent superior border of the pronator teres. The proximal radial shaft is then exposed by elevating the supinator subperiosteally, thus preserving the posterior interosseous nerve which rests between its two heads (Figure 12.18(b)). The pronator teres insertion should be respected or, if violated, carefully restored.

The radial canal containing the posterior interosseous

nerve can be released and explored, exposing the posterior interosseous nerve (up to its decussation into superficial and deep branches) by sequentially incising the fibrous band lying anterior to the radial head, the radial recurrent vessels as mentioned above, the surrounding fibrous margin of the extensor carpi radialis brevis, the arcade of Frohse and the entire superficial head of the supinator over the course of this nerve.

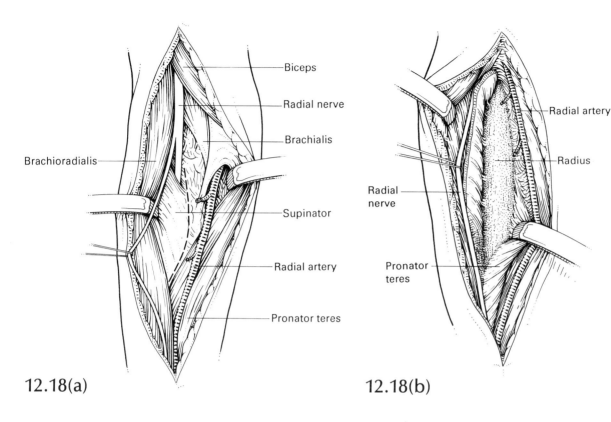

Biceps

Radial nerve

Brachialis

Brachioradialis

Supinator

Radial artery

Pronator teres

12.18(a)

Radial artery

Radius

Radial nerve

Pronator teres

12.18(b)

Indications

This approach is used to decompress or repair the distal radial nerve and particularly its deep posterior interosseous branch. It may also be used to reconstruct fractures, deformities, delayed unions or non-unions in the proximal third of the radial shaft. If a plate is used for such a repair, it must be secured with the forearm fully pronated, otherwise the plate will block pronation. This incision, combined with the anterior (Pheasant) incision to the elbow (see p. 169), may be used to approach the median nerve, if it is entrapped at the pronator or sublimis arch level. This incision may be extended the entire length of the forearm to expose either the median nerve or the radial artery for decompression, repair or reconstruction. The radial head, lateral elbow joint and capitellum can also be reached through this incision.

Posterolateral approach (Speed and Boyd)

Access

This incision gives exposure to the proximal third of the ulna and proximal fourth of the radius.

Position

The patient is supine with the shoulder abducted and internally rotated, the upper extremity being supported on an arm table with the elbow flexed and the forearm pronated.

Incision

The incision is started 2.5 cm above the elbow joint just lateral to the triceps tendon and extends distally over the olecranon and subcutaneous border of the proximal third of the ulna (Figure 12.19(a)).

Approach

Incise the deep fascia in line with the incision so as to approach the lateral border of the ulna between the anconeus insertion and the flexor carpi ulnaris (Figure 12.19(b)). The anconeus is reflected laterally after incising its ulnar insertion. This exposes the proximal third of the ulna on its lateral border and the supinator muscle (Figure 12.19(c)). The supinator can be incised near its ulnar origin and dissected subperiosteally to the interosseous membrane (Figure 12.19(c),(d)). The anconeus and supinator

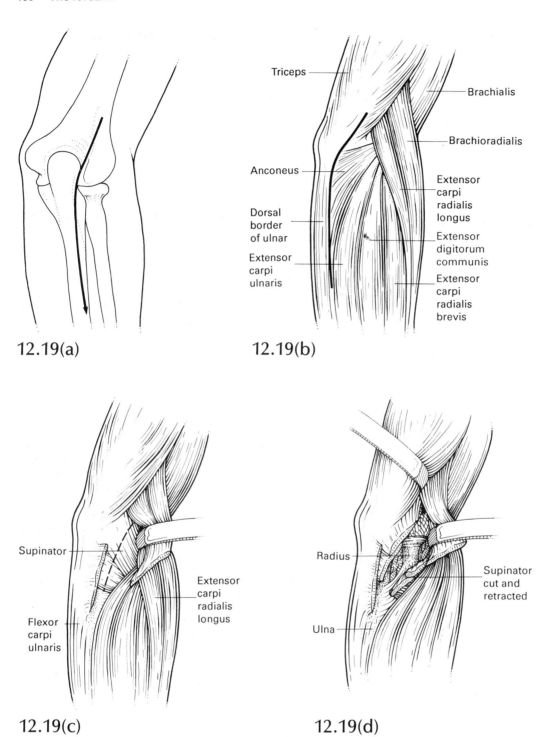

12.19(a)

12.19(b)

Triceps

Brachialis

Brachioradialis

Anconeus

Extensor carpi radialis longus

Dorsal border of ulnar

Extensor digitorum communis

Extensor carpi ulnaris

Extensor carpi radialis brevis

12.19(c)

Supinator

Extensor carpi radialis longus

Flexor carpi ulnaris

12.19(d)

Radius

Supinator cut and retracted

Ulna

are then freed from the posterior aspect of the interosseous membrane, carefully protecting the posterior interosseous nerve in the supinator substance. The anconeus and supinator are retracted radially to expose the posterior articular capsule over the radial head and the proximal fourth of the radius (Figure 12.19(d)). The recurrent interosseous artery is ligated and divided, but the posterior interosseous artery is preserved.

Indications

This approach is especially useful for treating fractures of the proximal ulna associated with radial head dislocations. It can be used for fractures, delayed unions and non-union of the proximal fourth of the ulna. It may also be used for fractures or dislocations of the radial head and neck with minimal risk of injury to the posterior interosseous nerve.

Posterolateral approach (Thompson)

Access

This approach provides access to the proximal two-thirds of the radius.

Position

The patient lies supine with the shoulder abducted and internally rotated. The upper extremity is supported on an arm table with the elbow flexed and the forearm pronated.

Incision

A straight skin incision is made over the proximal two-thirds of the radius on a line from the centre of the dorsum of the wrist to a point 1.5 cm anterior to the lateral humeral epicondyle with the forearm pronated (Figure 12.20(a)).

Approach

The incision is carried through the subcutaneous tissue and deep fascia, between the extensor carpi radialis brevis and the extensor digitorum communis (Figure 12.20(b)). The seam between these two muscles is split (Figure 12.20(c)) and they are retracted apart exposing the supinator (Figure 12.20(d)). Improved exposure may be obtained by detaching some or all of the extensor digitorum origin from the lateral humeral epicondyle. The insertion of the supinator onto the radius may be reflected medially, from distal to proximal, by subperiosteal dissection leaving the posterior interosseous nerve submerged and protected within its substance (Figure 12.20(d)). This is facilitated by supinating the forearm. The posterior interosseous nerve can be identified where it emerges at the inferior edge of the supinator (Figure 12.20(d)) or by intramuscular dissection in the mid-substance of the deep head and then by sufficient exposure to assure its protection (Figure 12.20(e)). The supinator and abductor pollicis longus are then gently retracted medially to expose the proximal two-thirds of the radius (Figure 12.20(f)).

Indications

This incision is useful for repair of acute fractures, delayed or ununited fractures, the removal of tumours or the clearance of infections in the proximal half of the radius. The posterior interosseous nerve can be explored through this incision for repair, decompression or reconstruction.

Anterodistal approach (Henry)

Access

This incision provides access to the anterior surface of the distal half of the radius.

Position

The patient lies supine with the shoulder abducted and externally rotated. The upper extremity is placed on an adjacent arm table with the elbow extended and the forearm supinated.

Incision

This incision is extensile with the more proximal anterior approach to the forearm (see p. 185). The incision starts at the flexion crease of the wrist and parallels the radial border of the flexor carpi radialis tendon between it and the brachioradialis for a distance of 15–20 cm (Figure 12.21(a)).

Approach

The subcutaneous tissue and deep fascia are incised in line with the skin incision. The radial artery is identified between the tendons of the brachioradialis and the flexor carpi radialis (Figure 12.21(b)). The sensory branch of the radial nerve is identified beneath the brachioradialis where it is protected and retracted laterally with the brachioradialis. The radial artery and its accompanying veins are retracted medially with the flexor carpi radialis, exposing from proximal to distal the flexor digitorum superficialis, the flexor pollicis longus and the pronator quadratus (Figure 12.21(c)). The forearm is then pronated to expose the border of the radius just lateral to the lateral edges of the flexor pollicis longus and the pronator quadratus. The periosteum of the radius is then incised in line with the lateral borders of the flexor pollicis longus and the pronator quadratus (Figure 12.21(d)). These muscles are then reflected medially and the forearm is then supinated to expose the anterior border of the distal third to half of the radial shaft (Figure 12.21(e)).

Indications

This approach is suitable for acute fracture repair, repair of delayed union or non-union, corrective osteotomies, tumours or infections and repair of bone defects in the distal half of the radius.

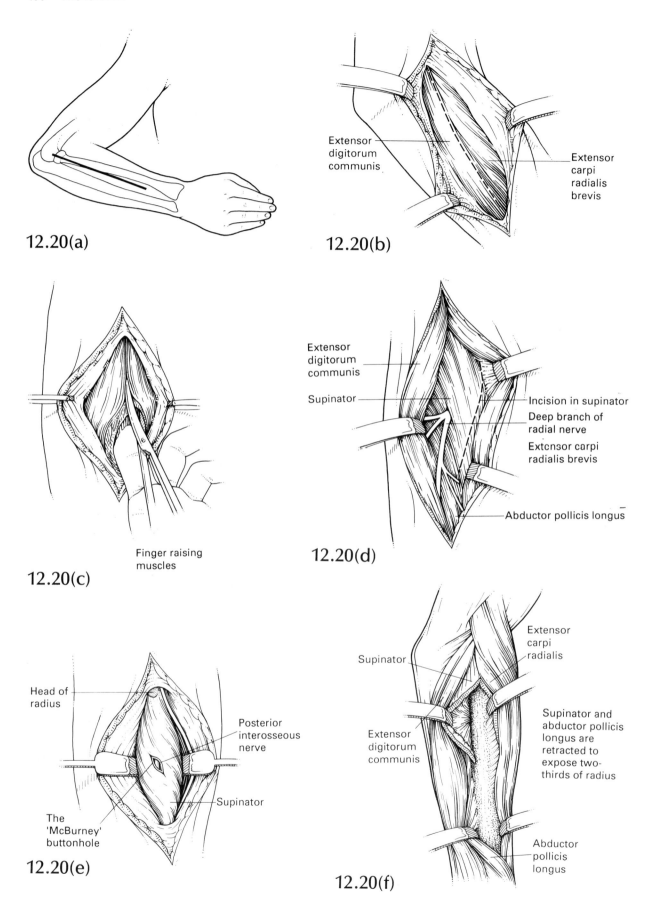

12.20(a)

12.20(b)

Extensor digitorum communis

Extensor carpi radialis brevis

Finger raising muscles

12.20(c)

Extensor digitorum communis

Supinator

Incision in supinator

Deep branch of radial nerve

Extensor carpi radialis brevis

Abductor pollicis longus

12.20(d)

Head of radius

Posterior interosseous nerve

The 'McBurney' buttonhole

Supinator

12.20(e)

Supinator

Extensor carpi radialis

Extensor digitorum communis

Supinator and abductor pollicis longus are retracted to expose two-thirds of radius

Abductor pollicis longus

12.20(f)

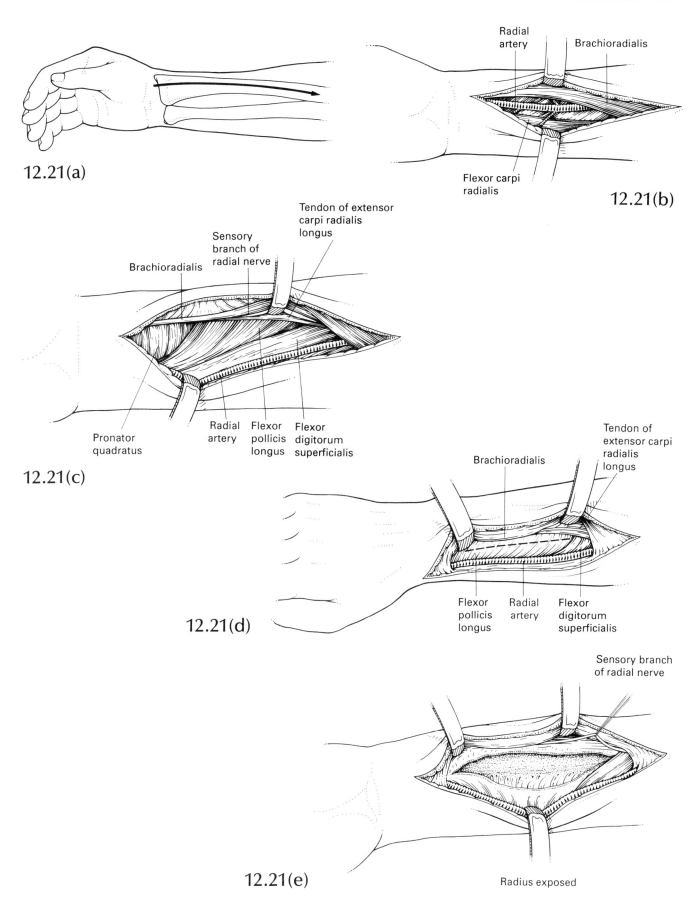

12.21(a)

12.21(b)
Radial artery
Brachioradialis
Flexor carpi radialis

12.21(c)
Brachioradialis
Sensory branch of radial nerve
Tendon of extensor carpi radialis longus
Pronator quadratus
Radial artery
Flexor pollicis longus
Flexor digitorum superficialis

12.21(d)
Brachioradialis
Tendon of extensor carpi radialis longus
Flexor pollicis longus
Radial artery
Flexor digitorum superficialis

12.21(e)
Sensory branch of radial nerve
Radius exposed

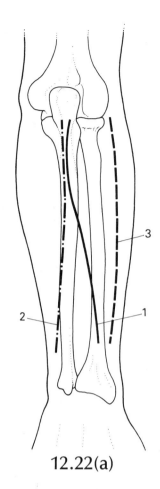

12.22(a)

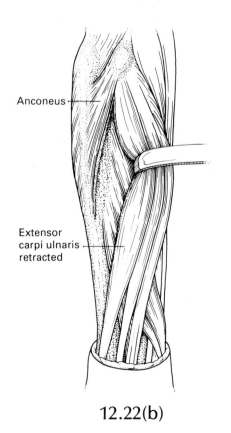

Anconeus

Extensor
carpi ulnaris
retracted

12.22(b)

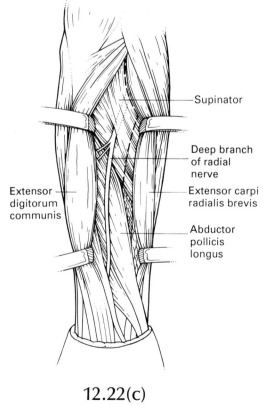

Extensor
digitorum
communis

Supinator

Deep branch
of radial
nerve

Extensor carpi
radialis brevis

Abductor
pollicis
longus

12.22(c)

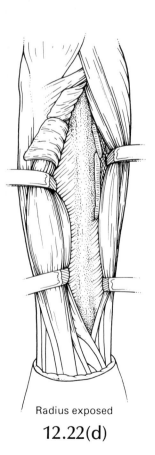

Radius exposed

12.22(d)

Combined posterior approach to the radius and ulna

Access

The proximal third of the ulnar shaft and the proximal two-thirds of the radial shaft can be approached simultaneously using a single incision. By using separate linear longitudinal incisions axially placed, the entirety of the ulnar shaft and the proximal two-thirds of the radial shaft can be exposed.

Position

The patient is supine on the operating table. The arm is abducted and positioned on an adjacent table with the elbow flexed and the forearm supinated.

Incision

A single incision may be used to approach simultaneously the proximal third of the ulnar shaft and the proximal two-thirds of the radial shaft, by starting proximally at the elbow between the olecranon and the lateral epicondyle and proceeding distally curving over the proximal third of the ulna and then back over the middle third of the radius (Figure 12.22(a): incision 1). If independent incisions are chosen, a linear longitudinal incision along the subcutaneous margin of the ulna is started 5 cm from the olecranon and extends as far as necessary towards the ulnar styloid (Figure 12.22(a): incision 2). A posterolateral (Thompson) approach is then used to expose the proximal two-thirds of the radius (Figure 12.22(a): incision 3).

Approach

The subcutaneous tissue and deep fascia are incised in line with the incision or incisions. When a single incision is used a full thickness skin and subcutaneous fat flap must be mobilized. To expose the shaft of the ulna, the periosteum is incised along the subcutaneous margin of the bone and the extensor carpi ulnaris is stripped laterally (Figure 12.22(b)). To expose the upper two-thirds of the radial shaft, the seam is split between the extensor carpi radialis brevis and the extensor digitorum communis exposing the supinator (Figure 12.22(c)). The approach is the same as the posterolateral (Thompson) approach (see p. 189). The deep posterior interosseous nerve is identified and visualized sufficiently to assure its protection and then the supinator is divided longitudinally over the lateral aspect of the radius and retracted medially with the extrinsic thumb muscles (Figure 12.22(d)). Using these approaches with either a single incision or with two incisions, concurrent fractures or lesions of the ulnar and radial shafts may be approached simultaneously.

Indications

This approach is used for the repair of recent fractures, reconstructions of delayed unions, non-unions and segmental bone loss, corrective osteotomies, benign or malignant tumours and bone infections of the ulnar shaft and the proximal two-thirds of the radial shaft.

References

Henry, A. K. (1973) *Extensile Exposure,* 2nd edn, Churchill Livingstone, Edinburgh, pp. 94–115
Speed, J. S. and Boyd, H. B. (1940) Treatment of fractures of the ulna with dislocation of the head of the radius (Monteggia fracture). *JAMA,* **115,** 1699
Thompson, J. E. (1918) Anatomical methods of approach in operations on the long bones of the extremities. *Ann. Surg.,* **68,** 309

Further reading

Boyd, H. B. (1940) Surgical exposure of the ulna and proximal third of the radius through one incision. *Surg. Gynecol. Obstet.,* **71,** 86
Henry, A. K. (1927) *Exposures of Long Bones and Other Surgical Methods,* John Wright, Bristol

Chapter 13

The wrist and hand

N. J. Barton

Introduction

The hand is a complex organ of irregular shape and packed with anatomical structures lying close together, so the surgical approaches cannot be classified as conveniently as in other chapters in this book.

The approach used will depend upon which anatomical structure, and how much of it, needs to be exposed. In general, transverse incisions, parallel to the skin creases, leave the least conspicuous scars (Boyes, 1962) and are therefore preferable if access is needed to only a limited area, as in operations for stenosing tenovaginitis or ganglia. However, most of the major structures run longitudinally and if they are to be exposed over some length, then an essentially longitudinal incision is better.

The words 'essentially longitudinal' are used because such incisions must not run across the flexion creases of the fingers lest subsequent contracture of the scar causes a flexion deformity (which may be just what the operation was intended to avoid or correct). This can be avoided in three ways (Figure 13.1):

1. A stepped, or bayonet, incision which incorporates one or more transverse incisions, preferably in flexion creases; sometimes there is no choice about this because the transverse wound may have already been created by the injury which has led to the operation. From one end of the transverse incision a longitudinal incision extends proximally, and from the other end a longitudinal incision extends distally (Figure 13.1(a)).
2. The incision may be made in a zig-zag shape, especially in the digits, so that it crosses the flexion creases at an angle, preferably out towards the end of the crease at the mid-lateral line (Figure 13.1(b)).
3. A straight incision is made, but before closure is broken up by one or more Z-plasties (not to be

confused with the initially zig-zag incision described above). The principles and techniques of Z-plasty are clearly and fascinatingly explained in McGregor's book *Fundamental Techniques of Plastic Surgery*. Essentially, what Z-plasty does is to gain length at the expense of width. There is little width to spare in the finger but, fortunately, if one makes several small Z-plasties in series (Figure 13.1(c)), the lengthening effect is cumulative, whereas the narrowing effect is not. Scars crossing the flexion creases in the palm, as opposed to the creases in the fingers or at the junction of finger and palm, do not usually result in flexion contractures and are, in my opinion, acceptable, though not all would agree with this.

Scar contracture seems to be largely a problem of the skin itself and not of the subcutaneous and deeper tissues. Once an incision has been made in the skin and properly developed, further incision into the deeper tissues can be made in any desired direction (Boyes, 1952).

Other considerations in planning the incision are the extent to which it must pass from one region into another, e.g. from the palm into the thumb, and the presence of open wounds or old scars. These are often present where the operation follows an injury, or may date from previous unsuccessful surgery. It is usually best to incorporate the earlier wound or scar into the new incision and this gives the opportunity to excise the scar if it is hypertrophic. However, it may be decided to ignore an old scar completely and make a new elective incision, provided this will not compromise the blood supply distal to the old scar. For the same reason, parallel wounds should not be too close together.

The more complex tendon transfer operations require access to many different parts of the hand, and the best solution is to use multiple small incisions. Some of these, such as those through which a tendon will be detached or

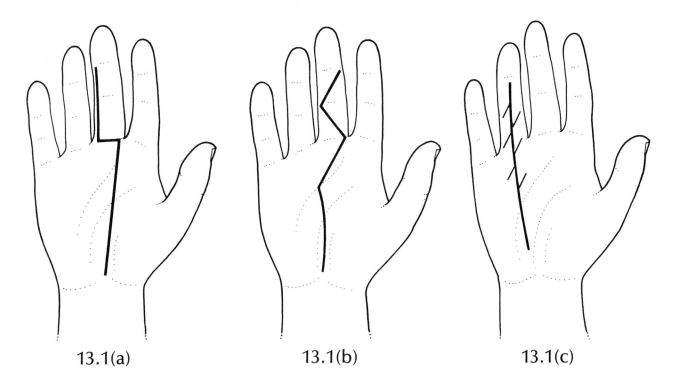

13.1(a)   13.1(b)   13.1(c)

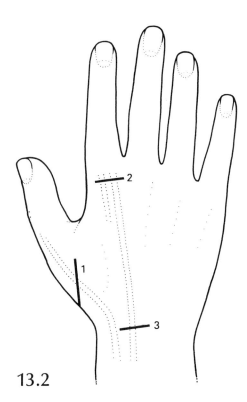

13.2

re-routed, can be tranverse (Figure 13.2), which causes the least possible scarring along the gliding surface of the tendon (Boyes, 1962) as well as the least conspicuous scar.

The cosmetic effect of scars on the hand must not be forgotten. The hands and face are the only parts of the body which are normally exposed to everyone and as the hand is put forwards in greeting or to give or receive something, a conspicuous scar is noticeable. As has been said, scars are less likely to become hypertrophic if they are parallel to the creases of the skin, most of which are transverse on both the front and the back of the hand. The palmar and volar finger creases are areas in which there is little or no subcutaneous fat, and it is better to be able to suture skin with subcutaneous tissue, so incisions should be parallel and close to a crease rather than in the crease itself (Boyes, 1962).

From the above considerations it will be seen that careful thought and planning are necessary and the wise surgeon will draw the incision on the skin, using a sterile marking pen, before picking up the scalpel. This gives the chance to see how it looks and to alter the angles or make other changes without doing any damage.

Figure 13.2 An example of multiple incisions for tendon transfer, in this case one of the simplest and most common transfers: that of extensor indicis proprius to extensor pollicis longus. Incision 1 is to expose the tendon of extensor pollicis longus distal to the point of rupture. To avoid having the scar along the line of the tendon (which runs obliquely), the incision is made longitudinally. Incision 2 is transverse, just proximal to the extensor hood. The extensor indicis proprius tendon is, contrary to what one might expect, the more ulnar of the two. This tendon is then put under tension so that it can be felt on the back of the wrist, where a transverse incision (3) is made through which the tendon can, after being detached, be re-routed towards the thumb

Surgical approaches

- Palmar fascia
    Transverse incision
    Essentially longitudinal incision
    Combinations of incisions
- Flexor tendons and median nerve
    Carpal tunnel exposure
    Extension above wrist
    Flexor tendons in fingers and thumb
        Mid-lateral incision
        Zig-zag incisions
- Extensor tendons
- Carpus
    Dorsal
    Radial
    Anterior

Palmar fascia

In the Western world, one of the most common disorders of the hand requiring surgery is Dupuytren's contracture. There is, however, no standard operation for this condition, because there is no standard pattern of disease. The incision must, therefore, be planned individually for each patient.

Most of the complications after fasciectomy relate to the early, and often widespread, attachment of the diseased tissue to the skin. Before planning the incision, the surgeon must decide:

(a) where there is diseased fascia, and
(b) where it is attached to skin.

It is suggested that a drawing be made in the clinical record (Figure 13.3) on which all palpable thickened fascia is marked by heavy shading, and all pits and other points of skin involvement marked by circles. The incision should, as far as possible, pass through the points of skin attachment so that these thinnest parts of the skin flaps which will be raised are at their edge and not in their base.

The pattern of disease will determine whether the incision is essentially transverse, essentially longitudinal, or a combination of both.

Transverse incision

If the disease is confined mainly to the palm, a transverse incision in, or close to, the distal palmar crease gives good access.

Since it passes along a watershed in the cutaneous blood supply, it should not interfere with the vascularity of the flaps, but in practice it was found that, if a radical palmar fasciectomy was performed and the wound sutured, many complications arose. For this reason that procedure is not favoured today. If a transverse cut is used, it should be left wide open, as described by McCash (1964). After correction of the contracture, there may be a

gap of up to 2 cm between the skin edges, but there is no skin missing and it is amazing how, as the wound heals, the skin edges are drawn together to produce a linear scar over 4–6 weeks. Lubahn, Lister and Wolfe (1984) have shown that better results are obtained by this technique.

Some surgeons also use a transverse incision, left open, in the finger at the basal flexion crease and/or the proximal interphalangeal flexion crease. This gives only very limited access and is more suitable for open fasciotomy than for fasciectomy.

Essentially longitudinal incision

If the disease is distributed longitudinally, from the palm into the finger, then an essentially longitudinal incision gives the best exposure. However, as discussed earlier, this must be modified in some way to avoid a straight longitudinal scar, at least in the finger. In the palm, scar contracture is seldom a problem and a gently sinuous incision is satisfactory.

1. Straight incision with Z-plasties (Figure 13.4)

A straight incision is made down the mid-line of the finger. The diseased cord is usually inserted onto the fibrous flexor sheath at the base of the middle phalanx, so the incision needs to go at least as far as the centre of the middle phalanx (McFarlane (1988) always takes it to the

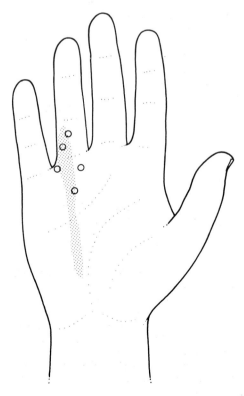

13.3

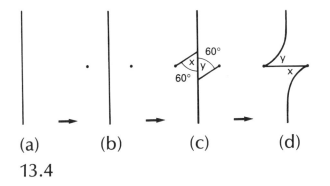

(a)   (b)   (c)   (d)

13.4

than with any other, and therefore uses it routinely in milder cases, but if the contractures are severe it is preferable to use Z-plasties which actually lengthen the scar.

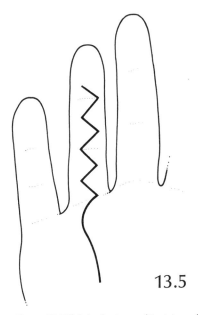

13.5

Figure 13.5 This is the type of incision which the author has found most useful and least troublesome in operations for Dupuytren's contracture. The fact that it crosses the palmar creases does not seem to give rise to contracture or other problems (provided it does not cross a transverse palmar incision which is left open to heal slowly: the McCash technique): however, it certainly must not run straight across the flexion creases of the finger

distal flexion crease). The Z-plasties should not be made until the end of the operation, when it can be seen where the skin is thinnest, so that any very thin skin is at the edge, rather than at the base, of any flap.

Deepen the incision to the diseased tissue. In some places it will be possible to preserve a thick layer of skin and fat, whereas in others the disease is close beneath the skin, which therefore ends up very thin, effectively a full-thickness graft. The skin should be handled gently with a fine skin hook and *never* with forceps which would further damage it.

Before closure, mark two spots about 7 mm on each side of the incision and opposite each other (Figure 13.4(b)). If these can be located in the flexion creases it is an advantage, but it is more important to make flaps in well-vascularized skin. Draw parallel lines joining each spot to the incision at an angle of 60 degrees (Figure 13.4(c)). Holding what is going to be the apex with a skin hook, cut along this line through skin and fat to form a triangular flap. Avoid cutting too deeply and damaging the neurovascular bundle of the finger. Transpose the flaps. If this is done correctly, they should lie in their transposed position without any difficulty. Suture the apices, and insert a few other fine stitches as necessary. It is best not to suture the transverse limb but to leave it open like a 'McCash': this diminishes both tension and the risk of haematoma.

2. Zig-zag incision

The larger zig-zag described by Bruner (1973) will be described in the approach to flexor tendons (see p. 202).

For Dupuytren's, the smaller zig-zag described by Hiles (1983) is recommended, as the incision stays closer to the longitudinal line of the disease and the skin flaps are smaller (Figure 13.5). The sides should be about 1 cm long and the angle 90 degrees or slightly less. The incision should be arranged so that the parts which cross the flexion creases coincide with one of the angles. There will, of course, also be angles in between these creases. Preferably using magnification, the diseased collagen bundles are carefully dissected off the skin as far as the subdermal vascular plexus, which should be preserved. Closure should be with stitches at the apices only, to allow free drainage of any blood.

The author has had fewer problems with this incision

3. Mid-lateral incision

This does not usually give satisfactory access to Dupuytren's disease, but a partially mid-lateral approach may be useful in two of the less common types of Dupuytren's contracture.

The first type is that disease which arises from the fascia over the abductor digiti minimi and passes along the ulnar border of the little finger (Barton, 1984). If sought, this is present in most cases of contracture of the little finger, and the approach should *always* allow a view of the insertion of abductor digiti minimi. Conversely, where the disease is obviously on the ulnar side of the finger it is wise to have at least one Hiles zig-zag to expose the palmar aspect in order to give access to any disease coming from the palm (Figure 13.6).

The second type is the corresponding, but rarer, disease on the side of one of the other fingers, arising from the fascia over one of the interosseous muscles (Strickland and Bassett, 1985). In this situation, the mid-lateral incision can be continued into the palm by curving into the web (Figure 13.7) so that it does not cross the basal flexion crease of the finger (Carr, 1974).

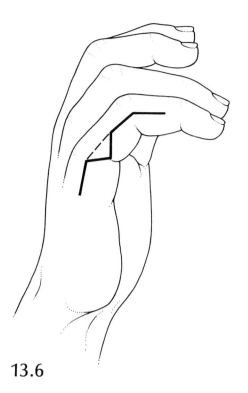

13.6

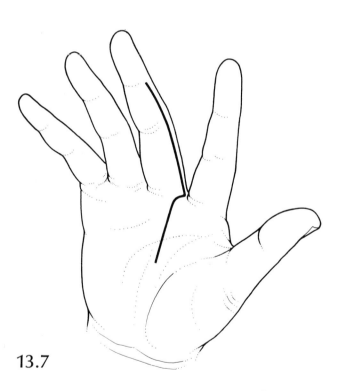

13.7

Combinations of incisions

The most difficult problems arise when more than one finger is involved, and it is necessary to plan an incision combining elements of those described above.

The main concern is to preserve a blood supply to the distal skin flap between two longitudinal incisions. One solution is not to incise that part of skin, but to tunnel subcutaneously from the palmar incision to the base of the finger. This is distasteful and risky, because one cannot see the digital nerve and vessel (which may be displaced by the disease process at the base of the finger), but for an experienced surgeon can be a satisfactory solution if done with great care.

Alternatively, the longitudinal incisions for two fingers may join a transverse palmar incision. If this is done, the distal flap between them should be as broadly based as possible, and the transverse incision should definitely *not* be sutured. Any longitudinal incision made in the proximal part of the palm must not join the transverse palmar incision opposite the distal longitudinal incision, or a continous longitudinal incision will result and this is very likely to cause a contracture when combined with the 'open palm' technique of McCash, which depends upon contracture for healing.

Flexor tendons and median nerve

A limited exposure suitable for the release of a trigger finger or thumb can be obtained by a transverse incision placed, not over a skin crease, but over what is judged to be the proximal end of the fibrous flexor sheath, usually about 2 cm proximal to the basal flexor crease. If there is more than one trigger finger, the skin incision can be extended to cover both. In the fingers, the digital nerves lie on each side of the flexor tendon, but it is very important to remember that in the thumb both digital nerves lie anteriorly, almost in front of the flexor tendon.

The fullest exposure of the flexor tendons is needed for flexor tenosynovectomy and flexor tendon grafting. Parts of this approach are used to expose the flexor tendons for other purposes, or to decompress the median nerve.

It is easiest, though it may seem illogical, first to describe the central part of the approach and then work towards the ends.

EXPOSURE OF THE CARPAL TUNNEL

Anatomy

As far as surface anatomy is concerned, the flexor retinaculum is in the hand, not the wrist. It extends from the distal flexion crease of the wrist to the proximal end of the hollow in the centre of the palm. The flexor retinaculum is attached at its four corners to the pisiform, the hamate, the tuberosity of the scaphoid and the ridge of the trapezium (Figure 13.8). All these can be palpated before starting an operation, and the incision must obviously be a longitudinal one lying between the medial and lateral margins of the retinaculum.

An incision in this area can endanger the palmar cutaneous branch of the median nerve (Figure 13.8). Although this is a small nerve, damage to it may result in

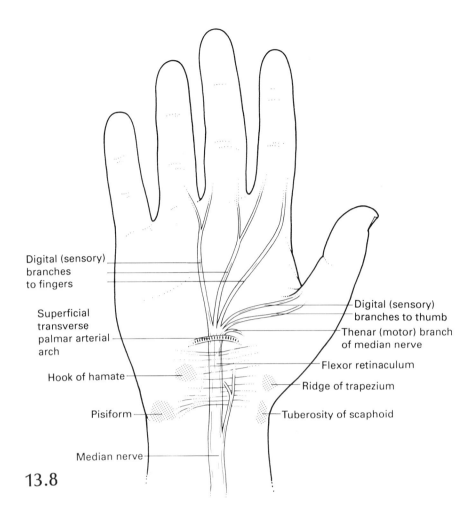

Digital (sensory) branches to fingers

Superficial transverse palmar arterial arch

Hook of hamate

Pisiform

Median nerve

Digital (sensory) branches to thumb

Thenar (motor) branch of median nerve

Flexor retinaculum

Ridge of trapezium

Tuberosity of scaphoid

13.8

painful hyperaesthesia in the palm, which in some cases is so severe that it prevents anything being held in the hand. This branch usually arises from the radial side of the main median nerve, 3–6 cm above the wrist, and runs close to the tendon of flexor carpi radialis. It nearly always lies to the radial side of the mid-line of the wrist (Das and Brown, 1976), so incisions in this area should be in the mid-line or slightly to the ulnar side.

Procedure

Identify the mid-point of the distal flexion crease of the wrist. Draw a line running from that point distally for 4 cm, which should carry you 'over the hill' and down into the central hollow of the palm (Figure 13.9(a)). The incision must *not* be radial to this, in order to avoid the palmar cutaneous nerve. The origins of the thenar muscles sometimes extend across to the ulnar side of the mid-line, so there is an advantage if the incision lies a few millimetres to the ulnar side of the mid-line; however, it must not go as far medially as the line of the hook of the hamate, which represents the ulnar limit of the carpal tunnel. It should, in fact, point roughly to the web between the middle and ring fingers.

There is no need studiously to follow skin creases, and a straight longitudinal incision is probably best, but, if there

is a convenient crease between the planned straight incision and the mid-line, then it may be followed.

Having made the skin incision, you may cut boldly down, through the insertion of the palmaris longus, until you reach the flexor retinaculum. A small, self-retaining retractor can be inserted to part the skin and fat.

The retinaculum is incised longitudinally with caution (Figure 13.9(b)), deepening the cut 1 mm at a time, in the same place, until the carpal tunnel is entered. This is enlarged just enough to admit the curved end of a MacDonald's dissector, which is passed distally while keeping its tip as superficial in the tunnel as possible. As it is introduced, the dissector must be lifted to press closely against the deep surface of the flexor retinaculum so that it is kept superficial to the superficial palmar arch (Figure 13.8): division of this superficial arch does not cause ischaemia, but it does cause a haematoma. Cut down through the flexor retinaculum onto the dissector until you can see that you have reached the distal end of the retinaculum. Take out the dissector, reintroduce it the other way (going proximally) and complete the division of the retinaculum which suddenly thins out to become the deep fascia of the forearm.

Indication

Decompression of the carpal tunnel.

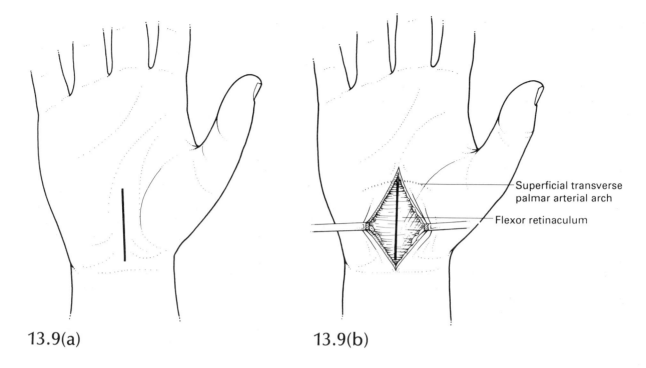

13.9(a)   13.9(b)

Superficial transverse palmar arterial arch

Flexor retinaculum

EXTENSION ABOVE THE WRIST OF CARPAL TUNNEL EXPOSURE (p. 198)

Procedure

Introduce a step into the incision, by incorporating a short transverse incision in the distal flexion crease of the wrist, and then continue proximally (Figure 13.10). If there is already a transverse wound or scar, that is incorporated instead of making a new one. This should usually be to the ulnar side of the mid-line, partly to avoid damage to the palmar cutaneous nerve of the median nerve, but also because the long digital flexors lie in the ulnar two-thirds of the front of the wrist.

Indications

Repair of cut nerves and tendons. Flexor tenosynovectomy (e.g. rheumatoid). Carpal tunnel syndrome following a Colles' fracture. Certain flexor tendon reconstructions, e.g. tendon graft to the thumb, or implantation of a silastic rod.

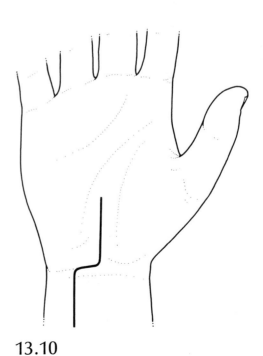

13.10

FLEXOR TENDONS IN THE FINGERS AND THUMB

Anatomy

There are three flexion creases in each finger and two in the thumb which must be circumnavigated, as discussed in the introduction to this chapter, to avoid the development of a subsequent contracture. Obviously, it is also necessary to avoid injury to the digital nerves and vessels. The unique problems of the digital flexor tendons stem from the combination of their lengthy excursion and their location in thick fibrous sheaths which are attached to the flat anterior surfaces of the phalanges. Any adhesions which may form after injury or operation will fix the flexor tendon to inelastic structures and limit active flexion of the digit.

There is no escaping the need to incise the tendon sheath, but current thought favours incision rather than excision, raising the sheath as a flap, which is then either allowed to fall back into place, or carefully sutured under the operating microscope if this can be done without causing any constriction. Broadly speaking, the anterior half of the finger (Figure 13.11(a)) is occupied by the flexor tendons in their sheath, covered by subcutaneous fat. The posterior half is occupied by the phalanx, on which lies dorsally a thin sheet of extensor tendon. The digital arteries and nerves are not quite in the mid-lateral line, but slightly anterior to it, with the nerve lying in front of the artery.

In the thumb (Figure 13.11(b)), the nerves and vessels are not mid-lateral at all, but definitely anterior; one nerve may even lie partly in front of the flexor tendon sheath.

Approaches

If the incision is to avoid crossing the flexion creases, then it must pass posterior to the ends of these creases. The choice is whether to continue to the end of the next crease on the same side of the finger (a mid-lateral incision) as in Figure 13.12(a), or to cross the finger obliquely to the end of the next crease on the other side (Bruner zig-zag incision) as in Figure 13.13(a). The number of zigs depends on the length of the segment; the variability of this incision is one of its advantages. In the case of injuries, there will already be a transverse, or oblique, cut which may be followed to the other side of the finger. Electively, a zig-zag series of oblique incisions may be made. The advantages of the mid-lateral incision, which was used by the pioneers of hand surgery, are that it avoids scarring the precious anterior skin, and that it is easier to close with the finger flexed (Littler, 1974). In practice, however, a scar on the palmar surface (if properly designed) does not cause problems and it is not necessary to maintain much flexion while suturing the skin. The disadvantage is that the exposure is not so good and the mid-lateral incision is now less popular. Most prefer a zig-zag type of incision, but both are described here, as special circumstances may favour one or the other.

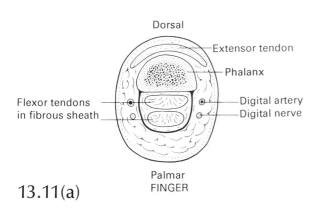

13.11(a)

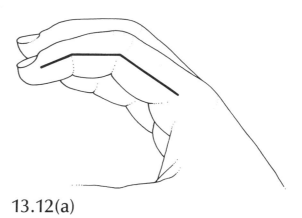

13.12(a)

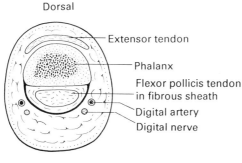

13.11(b)

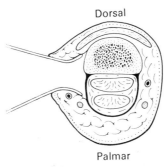

13.12(b)

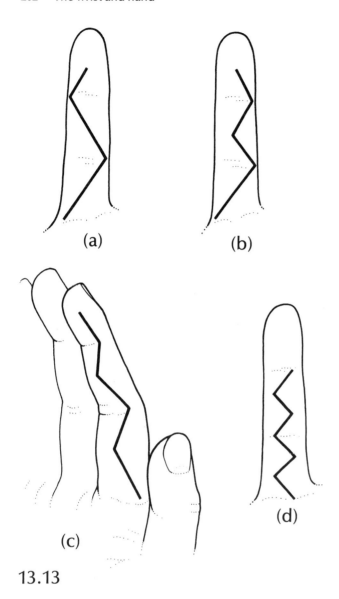

(a)   (b)

(c)

(d)

13.13

on the anterior flap, leaving the neurovascular bundle *in situ* and exposing the tendon sheath *in front of it*; but this method is not widely used.

Incise the fibrous sheath longitudinally, enough to expose the area of flexor tendon to which access is needed. It will be necessary also to incise the sheath transversely at one or both ends of the longitudinal incision in order to raise a flap of sheath which will give a good view of the tendon, but if those thick sections of sheath which form the pulleys have not already been damaged by injury they should be preserved (Lister, 1983).

Zig-zag incisions

The large zig-zag incision, described by Bruner (1973) and shown in Figures 13.1(b), and 13.13(a), gives good access to the flexor tendon sheath and to the digital nerve and artery, but care must be taken not to damage these structures while raising or suturing the angles of the flap.

Various other forms of zig-zag incisions have also been described, all of which give better access to a narrower strip down the finger:

1. The 'W' incision of Littler (1974) shown in Figure 13.13(b).
2. The lateral zig-zag (Hall and Vliegenthart, 1986), which is really a modified mid-lateral incision (Figure 13.13(c)). The neurovascular bundles remain with the *dorsal* flap as favoured by Rank, Wakefield and Hueston (1973).
3. The small zig-zag of Hiles, which has already been described (p. 197) and which is illustrated in Figure 13.13(d).

Indications

Repair of cut flexor tendons. Tendon grafting. Flexor tenosynovectomy. Tumours involving the flexor tendons, e.g. pigmented villonodular synovitis.

Mid-lateral incision

The ulnar side is preferable. On the index finger, the temptation to use the more accessible radial side should be resisted as this side of the finger is so important in fine manipulations and key grip that it should be left unscarred.

Draw a line along the side of the finger joining the ends of the flexion creases (Figure 13.12(a)). Cut down in this line until you reach the side of the flexor tendon sheath, close to its attachment to the phalanx (Figure 13.12(b)). Retract the skin and fat anteriorly, using a small blunt hook, with great care as this flap contains the digital nerve and artery, neither of which should be stretched or damaged in any way.

Rank, Wakefield and Hueston (1973), having made the skin incision as described, advocated elevating only skin

Extensor tendons

The skin on the back of the hand is lax and elastic so as to allow full flexion, and scar contracture is hardly ever a problem. It is therefore not necessary to make stepped or even sinuous incisions. What may be a problem, especially in rheumatoid patients, is getting the skin to heal, and most experienced surgeons have found that the least problems are encountered after straight longitudinal incisions.

The extensor tendons are not far beneath the skin and the only other significant structure which may need to be divided to expose them is the extensor retinaculum. Before incising the retinaculum, the surgeon must decide what to do with it at the end of the operation, as that will determine where and how it is incised.

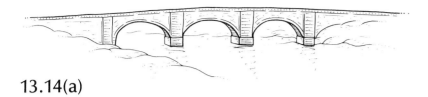

13.14(a)

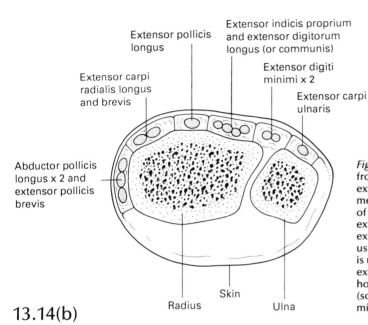

Extensor pollicis longus

Extensor indicis proprium and extensor digitorum longus (or communis)

Extensor carpi radialis longus and brevis

Extensor digiti minimi x 2

Extensor carpi ulnaris

Abductor pollicis longus x 2 and extensor pollicis brevis

Skin

Radius

Ulna

13.14(b)

Figure 13.14 Cross-section of wrist showing the septa running from the extensor retinaculum down to the bones dividing the extensor surface up into six compartments, like the piers of a mediaeval bridge. The compartments contain different numbers of tendons. There is, of course, more than one tendon for extensor digitorum longus (formerly and more sensibly called extensor digitorum communis), although at this level there are usually three, rather than four, because the one to the little finger is usually just a branch, over the distal metacarpal, from the extensor digitorum longus tendon to the ring finger. In addition, however, abductor pollicis longus has at least two tendons (sometimes three and occasionally four) and abductor digiti minimi usually has two small ones

Anatomy

The extensor retinaculum is not a single-span bridge across the tendons. It is more like a mediaeval bridge with many short spans: between these, septa pass down from the retinaculum to the underlying bone (Figure 13.14), forming six compartments containing varying numbers of tendons (Palmer *et al.*, 1985). A knowledge of the normal interconnections between the extensor tendons on the backs of the metacarpals, especially those involving the extensor tendon to the ring finger, is important. If you put your hand flat on a table, palm down, and extend each finger in turn as far as you can, you will find that the ring finger extends the least. Whereas the extensor indicis proprius and the extensor digitorum longus to the index finger are both long separate tendons, the extensor digitorum longus to the little finger is usually just a short branch from the extensor digitorum longus tendon to the ring finger. The extensor digiti minimi, however, has two tendons. There is also a connecting slip from the extensor tendon of the ring finger to that of the middle finger. In the nineteenth century, it was fashionable for musicians to have these connecting slips surgically divided, to give them a greater range and independence of extension of the ring finger (Parrott and Harrison, 1980). Nowadays, they are regarded as useful because they may enable a patient to extend all the fingers even when one tendon is divided or ruptured. As they also help to prevent sideways displacement of the extensor tendons, they should be preserved whenever possible.

Approach

1. Make a straight longitudinal incision over that part of the extensor tendon which is to be exposed.
2. Cut down through the subcutaneous fat (ligating and dividing any veins encountered) until the tendon or retinaculum is reached, and then bluntly separate off the fat. It is important to keep the skin flap as thick and as well-vascularized as possible. Retraction must be very gentle, particularly in rheumatoid patients.
3. If only one compartment is to be opened, there is no problem, but if it is necessary to expose more than one group of tendons, the sagittal septa which hold down the retinaculum to the carpus, between each group of tendons, must be divided so that the retinaculum can be lifted up as a flap (Figure 13.15). Before so doing, it must be decided whether to leave the intact attachment of the retinaculum on the radial or ulnar side. The latter is to be preferred as the natural tendency of the tendons (except for extensor pollicis longus) is to displace to the ulnar side. While incising and elevating the extensor retinaculum, particular care is taken of extensor pollicis longus: first, it must not be cut (which is easy to do because it is running obliquely across the line of the other tendons), and secondly, one should preserve a small strip of retinaculum which can later be made into a pulley to keep the extensor pollicis longus tendon in place on the ulnar side of Lister's tubercle (Figure 13.16).

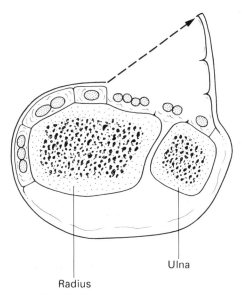

13.15

Radius

Ulna

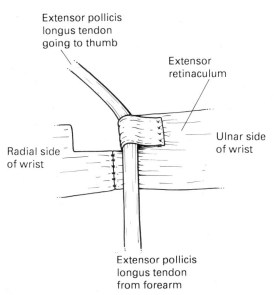

Extensor pollicis
longus tendon
going to thumb

Extensor
retinaculum

Radial side
of wrist

Ulnar side
of wrist

Extensor pollicis
longus tendon
from forearm

13.16

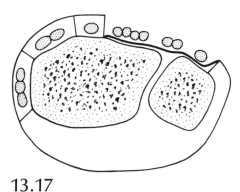

13.17

It is probably not good practice to suture the retinaculum over the extensor tendons, as this may cause a constriction, and certainly not in rheumatoid disease. Indeed, Savill argued that decompression is all that need be done for extensor tenosynovitis (Abernethy and Dennyson, 1979). It is probably wise in rheumatoid patients, especially if erosions have roughened the backs of the bones at the wrist, to replace the retinaculum *deep* to the tendons, in order to protect them from the underlying disease (Figure 13.17). Arthritic involvement of the wrist usually means that the range of wrist movement is limited, so 'bow-stringing' is not a problem. The retinacular dissection should be performed so as to raise it as a flap, based on the ulnar side, unless excision of the distal ulna is also planned, in which case a radially based retinacular flap is fashioned.

Indications

Access to the extensor tendons for any purpose. The most usual is tenosynovectomy for rheumatoid disease, or repair after trauma.

Carpus

Obviously the approach chosen will depend upon which area of the carpus is to be exposed. Ulnar approaches to the carpus are uncommon, because access to the hamate, triquetral and pisiform is seldom necessary.

The carpal bones are small, so the various joints are only a centimetre or two away from each other. It is surprisingly easy to mistake one bone or joint for another. It is therefore wise to expose the part and then confirm the site by sticking a needle into it and taking an X-ray, before proceeding to any definitive procedure. This applies particularly to the lunate. It should not be necessary for the trapezium, as the base of the first metacarpal is easily palpable and the saddle-joint, once opened, can be easily recognized.

DORSAL APPROACH

Technique

The skin incision may be transverse or longitudinal. If only limited access is required, as for a ganglion, a transverse incision leaves a less conspicuous scar. If the whole length of the carpus must be seen, then a longitudinal incision is necessary. It should be straight, not sinuous, especially in the thin skin of rheumatoid patients which may be very slow to heal at this site. Once through the skin, the approach must be longitudinal between the extensor tendons. The extensor retinaculum is divided longitudinally over the target area (unless it is planned to transpose it as a flap deep to the tendons, as described above, in which case it is divided to one or other side).

The extensor tendons are retracted with blunt hooks, exposing the dorsal capsule of the wrist joint.

If the operation is for a ganglion, then that part of the

capsule from which it arises must be excised together with the ganglion, or it will recur.

Angelides and Wallace (1976) have shown that the site of origin of dorsal wrist ganglia, wherever they may present on the surface, is the scapholunate joint, so to prevent recurrence it is always necessary to excise the capsule over that joint.

If the operation is on the carpal bones, the dorsal capsule is incised longitudinally over the part required, and then freed by sharp dissection on either side from its attachments to the underlying bones.

The usual mistake is to make the exposure more distal than intended, e.g. to expose the head of the capitate rather than the lunate. To avoid this, identify the radiocarpal joint by palpation before incising the capsule.

Indications

Excision of dorsal wrist ganglion. Operations on the lunate. Ligamentous reconstructions. Partial or complete arthrodesis.

RADIAL APPROACH

Anatomy

There are two important structures to avoid:

1. The superficial radial nerve, which may be in two separate parts, running parallel along the radial side of the wrist.
2. The radial artery, with its accompanying veins coming from the front of the radius, crosses the waist of the scaphoid on its radial side to pass dorsally to the space between the bases of the first and second metacarpals.

To cut the artery is careless and obvious, but a large haematoma may result from dividing one of its small branches whilst mobilizing the main artery in order to allow it to be retracted: these should therefore be identified and diathermied with a bipolar coagulator some distance from the main artery before they are divided.

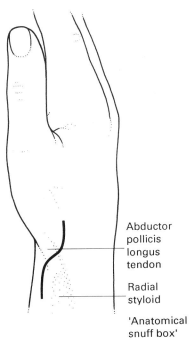

Abductor pollicis longus tendon

Radial styloid

'Anatomical snuff box'

13.18(a)

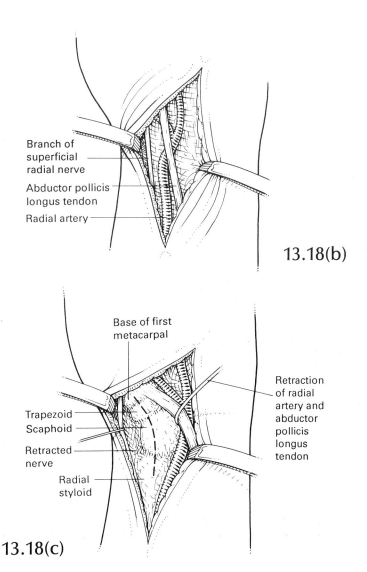

Branch of superficial radial nerve

Abductor pollicis longus tendon

Radial artery

13.18(b)

Base of first metacarpal

Retraction of radial artery and abductor pollicis longus tendon

Trapezoid
Scaphoid

Retracted nerve

Radial styloid

13.18(c)

Technique

The skin incision follows roughly the line of the radial artery, with a central oblique section as shown (Figure 13.18(a)). Take care not to cut the nerve with your skin incision.

Retract the nerve in whatever direction seems most helpful (Figure 13.18(b)). Coagulate and divide the anterior branches of the radial artery, which is then retracted dorsally (Figure 13.18(c)).

If necessary, partly detach the abductor pollicis longus from its insertion on the base of the first metacarpal.

Incise the capsule longitudinally.

Check that the carpal bone you have exposed is the one you want.

Indications

Excision of trapezium. Arthrodesis or arthroplasty of trapeziometacarpal joint. Exposure of distal pole of scaphoid, e.g. for internal fixation.

ANTERIOR APPROACH

The central part of the carpus is nearly always approached from the back, because it is nearer to the skin and the median nerve does not have to be retracted. The only exception is for open reduction of an anteriorly dislocated lunate or for reconstructions of the anterior ligaments (though the value of these is not proved). An anterior approach placed more laterally gives access to the scaphoid, as for bone grafting non-union. The classic description is that of Russe (1960), but this has been modified slightly by Herbert and Fisher (1984), whose approach will be described.

Technique

Incise the skin along the radial side of the distal 3 cm of the flexor carpi radialis tendon and then continue the incision distally across the distal wrist flexion crease, curving slightly radially along the line of the radially abducted first metacarpal (Figure 13.19(a)).

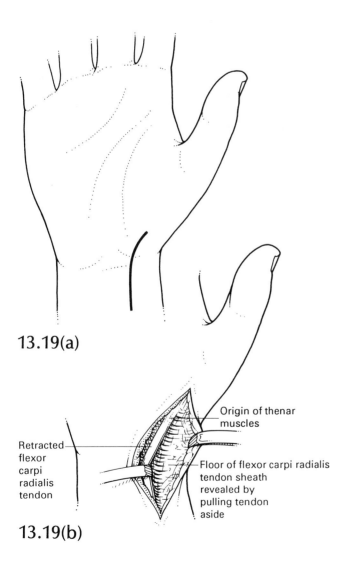

13.19(a)

Origin of thenar muscles

Retracted flexor carpi radialis tendon

Floor of flexor carpi radialis tendon sheath revealed by pulling tendon aside

13.19(b)

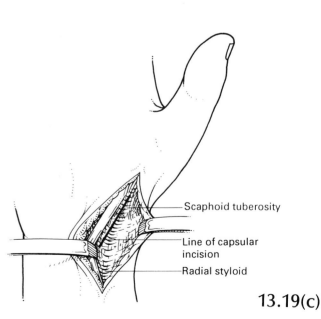

Scaphoid tuberosity

Line of capsular incision

Radial styloid

13.19(c)

Incise the radial side of the sheath of flexor carpi radialis and retract the tendon to the ulnar side (Figure 13.19(b)).

One or more small palmar branches of the radial artery may need to be ligated and divided.

Incise the floor of flexor carpi radialis tendon sheath: this is quite a thick, well-marked structure. Going through the middle of the bed of the tendon, rather than to its radial side, exposes the scaphoid a little further towards the ulnar side and gives a better view of its proximal pole. Deepen the incision to divide the anterior capsule of the wrist, in the line of the long axis of the scaphoid (Figure 13.19(c)), to expose the bone. The tuberosity protrudes anteriorly for a long way, whereas the waist and proximal pole are much deeper.

If a Herbert screw is to be inserted, the scaphotrapezial joint must be opened widely enough to fit the end of the jig onto the distal articular surface of the scaphoid. To expose this joint, the origin of the thenar muscles must be split for about 1 cm in the line of their fibres and retracted to either side.

Indication

Fractures of scaphoid requiring bone grafting and/or fixation with Herbert screw.

References

Abernethy, P. J. and Dennyson, W. G. (1979) Decompression of the extensor tendons at the wrist in rheumatoid arthritis. *J. Bone Joint Surg.*, **61B**, 64

Angelides, A. C. and Wallace, P. F. (1976) The dorsal ganglion of the wrist: its pathogenesis, gross and microscopic anatomy, and surgical treatment. *J. Hand Surg.*, **1**, 228

Barton, N. J. (1984) Dupuytren's disease arising from the abductor digiti minimi. *J. Hand Surg.*, **9B**, 265

Boyes, J. H. (1952) Operative technique in surgery of the hand. In *American Academy of Orthopaedic Surgeons Instructional Course Lectures*, vol. 9, C. V. Mosby, St Louis, pp. 181–195

Boyes, J. H. (1962) Incisions in the hand. *Am. J. Orthop.*, **4**, 308

Bruner, J. M. (1973) Surgical exposure of flexor tendons in the hand. *Ann. R. Coll. Surg. Engl.*, **53**, 84

Carr, T. L. (1974) Local radical fasciectomy for Dupuytren's contracture. *Hand*, **6**, 40

Das, S. K. and Brown, H. G. (1976) In search of complications of carpal tunnel decompression. *Hand*, **8**, 243

Hall, R. F. and Vliegenthart, D. H. (1986) A modified midlateral incision for volar approach to the digit. *J. Hand Surg.*, **11B**, 195

Herbert, T. J. and Fisher, W. E. (1984) Management of the fractured scaphoid using a new screw. *J. Bone Joint Surg.*, **66B**, 114

Hiles, R. W. (1983) Paper read at meeting of British Society for Surgery of the Hand, London, 11 November, 1983

Lister, G. D. (1983) Incision and closure of the flexor sheath during primary tendon repair. *Hand*, **15**, 123

Littler, J. W. (1974) Hand, wrist, and forearm incisions. In *Symposium on Reconstructive Hand Surgery* (eds J. W. Littler, L. H. Cramer and J. W. Smith), C. V. Mosby, St Louis, pp. 87–97

Lubahn, J. D., Lister, G. D. and Wolfe, T. (1984) Fasciectomy and Dupuytren's disease: a comparison between the open-palm technique and wound closure. *J. Hand Surg.*, **9A**, 53

McCash, C. R. (1964) The open palm technique in Dupuytren's contracture. *Br. J. Plast. Surg.*, **17**, 271

McFarlane, R. (1988) Dupuytren's contracture. In *Operative Hand Surgery*, vol. 1, 2nd edn (ed. D. P. Green), Churchill Livingstone, New York, pp. 553–589

McGregor, I. A. (1989) *Fundamental Techniques of Plastic Surgery*, 8th edn, Churchill Livingstone, Edinburgh

Palmer, A. K., Skahen, J. R., Werner, F. W. and Glisson, R. R. (1985) The extensor retinaculum of the wrist: an anatomical and biomechanical study. *J. Hand Surg.*, **10B**, 11

Parrott, J. R. and Harrison, D. B. (1980) Surgically dividing pianists' hands. *J. Hand Surg.*, **5**, 619

Rank, B. K., Wakefield, A. R. and Hueston, J. T. (1973) *Surgery of Repair as Applied to Hand Injuries*, 4th edn, Churchill Livingstone, Edinburgh

Russe, O. (1960) Fracture of the carpal navicular. Diagnosis, non-operative treatment and operative treatment. *J. Bone Joint Surg.*, **42A**, 759

Strickland, J. W. and Bassett, R. L. (1985) The isolated digital cord in Dupuytren's contracture: anatomy and clinical significance. *J. Hand Surg.*, **10A**, 118

Appendix of indications and their surgical approaches

Psoas tenotomy, 8, 22
Pubic ramus, fracture, 11
Pubic symphysis, disruption of, 11

Radial artery, decompression, 187
Radial head, dislocation, 169, 188
Radial nerve,
    decompression, 187
    exposure, 154, 155
Radius,
    bone defects, 189
    exposure of, 187
    fractures, 169, 187, 188, 189, 193
    infections, 189, 193
    non-union of fractures, 189, 193
    reconstruction, 187
    shaft fracture, 187
    tumours, 189, 193
Rheumatoid disease, 96, 201, 204
Rotator cuff,
    decompression, 146
    exposure, 142
    repair, 142, 143

Sacro-iliac joint,
    dislocation, 10
    exposure, 10
    osteosynthesis, 10
    subluxation, 10
Scaphoid,
    exposure, 206
    fractures, 207
Sciatic nerve,
    exposure, 21
    lesions, 31
Septic arthritis, 8, 21, 138
Shoulder,
    fracture-dislocation, 140
    loose bodies in, 138
    recurrent anterior dislocation, 138
    recurrent dislocation, 138, 145
    recurrent posterior subluxation, 145
    replacement, 139
    reversed Bankart's operation, 145
    septic arthritis, 138
    synovectomy, 138
Sinus tarsi lesions, 78
Subacromial region, impingement lesions, 142
Supracondylar fracture, 29, 163
Supraspinatus, exposure, 142
Synovium, biopsy, 8

Talofibular ligament, exposure, 78

Talus,
    anterolateral dislocation, 78
    lesions of dome, 84, 87
    osteochondral fracture, 87
    osteochondritis, 84, 87
Tarsal tunnel decompression, 93
Tennis elbow, 169
Tenosynovectomy, 204
Thumb, tendon graft to, 201
Tibia,
    bone grafting, 65, 66
    compression fracture, 79
    distal lesions, 79
    exposure, 49
    fractures, 54, 64, 78, 79
    lesions of, 84
    non-union of fractures, 65
    osteotomy, 71
    posterior lip fracture, 81
    reconstruction, 84
    shaft fracture, 54, 79
    supramalleolar fracture, 79
    tumours, 54, 68
Tibial condyles, fractures, 54
Tibial malleolus, posteromedial fractures, 84
Tibial spine, fractures, 49
Tibiofibular ligament, repair of, 91
Trapeziometacarpal joint, arthrodesis or arthroplasty, 206
Trapezium, excision, 206
Triceps,
    avulsion, 165
    snapping, 165
    tendon transfer, 165
Trochanter,
    exposure, 22
    osteoid osteoma, 22

Ulna,
    fractures, 175, 188, 193
    infections, 193
    non-union of fractures, 193
    tumours, 193
Ulnar nerve,
    decompression, 175
    repair or reconstruction, 175

Volkmann's fracture, 81, 82

Wrist,
    arthrodesis, 205
    reconstruction of tendons, 205
Wrist ganglion, excision, 205

Index